Dash Diet Cookbook

Recipes And Guide To Lower Blood Pressure, Lose Weight And Maintain Optimum Health

JEAN SIMMONS

ISBN-13:978-1720881735

ISBN-10:1720881731

DEDICATION

For Cindy,

Pleasant memories, always!

TABLE OF CONTENTS

INTRODUCTION

DASH Diet And Health

One of the biggest risk factors to serious health complications is an uncontrolled high blood pressure. High blood pressure can lead to more serious health issues like heart attacks, strokes, sexual dysfunction, kidney diseases, eye damage, bone loss (osteoporosis) and diabetes. This is because when blood pressure is high, the blood exerts too much force on the arteries walls as it pumps. Normal /regular Blood pressure reads 120/80 mmHg; any reading higher than this is considered high blood pressure. Sadly, 1 in 3 Americans adults have high blood pressure and the higher your blood pressure, the higher your risk of health complications.

There is good news however; and that good news is that an elevated blood pressure can be brought down by making a few lifestyle changes. One of these crucial changes is our diet. The right diet will make significant impact on our blood pressure readings as well as aid weight loss. This is where the Dash diet comes in. The Dash diet is one of the best diets for our health. And that is no exaggeration. The United States Department of Agriculture (USDA) approved the Dash diet as the best eating plan for all Americans. Additionally, the U.S news, together with a panel of health experts, evaluated 40 diets. DASH diet came out tops in many categories. It was ranked the best diets overall, best weight loss diet, best diabetes diet, best diet for healthy living, best fast weight loss diet, best heart healthy diet, and the easiest diet to follow. Promoted by the National Heart, Lung, and Blood Institute, the Dash diet is also recommended by the National Kidney Foundation for people with kidney disease.

But what is this Dash diet? DASH is simply an acronym for Dietary Approaches to Stop Hypertension. DASH diet has been irrefutably proven to lower blood pressure significantly within 14 days! Since it is low in saturated fat, it helps to reduce the risk of heart disease and hypertension. It also promotes weight loss. DASH reduces the risk of type 2 diabetes, especially when combined with weight management. It is a healthy eating plan that works best for diabetes and heart health. As a matter of fact, if you want to be healthy, then the Dash diet is for you.

DASH Diet involves eating plenty of fruits and vegetables as well as whole grain, meat, fish, poultry, beans, nuts and low-fat dairy foods. It is a diet that emphasizes plant-based foods that are loaded with powerful nutrients like potassium, calcium, magnesium, and fiber. These nutrients improve the balance of electrolyte in the body, enabling it to flush out excess fluid that promotes high blood pressure. Additionally, these nutrients helps the blood vessels relax well; which reduces blood pressure. People who are obese or overweight do not have enough of these nutrients. But by following a Dash diet, they take in these nutrients and are thus able to overcome their obesity and generally feel better about themselves. Dash diet works for short-term weight loss as well as long-term one. In some cases however, exercises or further carbohydrate reduction may be required to expedite the weight loss process.

DASH Diet And Blood Pressure

Since the concept of the Dash diet is to bring down an elevated blood pressure, we need to understand what this is all about. The normal blood pressure reading of a non-stressed adult is 120/80 mmHg. Two forces, the systolic and the diastolic pressure, pump blood through our bodies. They are measured by reference to two different numbers. The systolic pressure represents the highest point of pressure that is measured while the heart beats or contracts. It is the higher of the two numbers (120). The diastolic pressure, the lower figure, (80) is measured when the heart is resting between beats. It represents the low point of your blood pressure. Blood pressure is usually measured in millimeters of mercury and recorded as mmHg.

According to research, after 8 weeks of following DASH diet, a decrease in systolic blood pressure of about 6 mm Hg was recorded, and an average decrease in diastolic blood pressure of about 3 mm Hg was also noted. Patients with hypertension observed an 11 mm Hg drop in systolic blood pressure and a 6 mm Hg drop in diastolic blood pressure. DASH diet has been severally proven to be exceptional beneficial to your heart and overall health.

However, if you are on medication, discuss with your doctor before going on a dash diet. You do not want anything to interfere with the effectiveness of your medication. And if you start to feel sick after a few days of your being on this diet, revert to your original diet and see your doctor immediately.

Other contributory factors to reduce high blood pressure

1. Increase physical activity

2. Drink alcohol moderately

3. Increase potassium intake

4. Maintain a healthy body weight

5. Reduce sodium (salt) intake

DASH Diet & Low Sodium

Some people's high blood pressure is caused by too much sodium intake. Thankfully, DASH diet is a low sodium diet that aims to reduce sodium consumption in two ways:

1. The Standard DASH diet plan which permits a daily intake of up to 2,300 milligrams (mg) of sodium.

2. The Dash diet Sodium which involves limiting daily sodium intake to 1,500 mg. (about 2/3 teaspoon).

However, most people are advised to limit their sodium intake to 2,300 mg or less per day. But you can make gradual changes and measure your progress. For instance, you could begin by limiting your daily sodium intake to 2,400 milligrams, which is about 1 teaspoon. After a while, seeing how your body has adjusted, you can reduce your daily intake of sodium to 1,500 milligrams, which is about 2/3 teaspoon. Do not forget to include sodium eaten in foods and food products as well as the ones you add at the table and the ones you cook with.

DASH Diet And Its Core Components

DASH diet is easy to follow, convenient and non- restrictive. You can get your daily meal from each and every food group, even carbs. The focus is to reduce intake of salty, sugary and fatty foods as much as possible.

Eat:

- More Fruits And Vegetables
- More Low Fat Or Non Fat Dairy
- More whole-grain foods
- More Nuts, Seeds and Legumes
- More Lean Proteins

Limit:

- Foods high in saturated fat, transfats and cholesterol.
- Sodium and red meats as well as sweets and sugary drinks.
- Alcohol to 2 or fewer drinks everyday for men & 1 or less drink daily for women.

Eating such foods such as salads and Greek yoghurts, as well as snacks such as raw unsalted nuts, fruits and black bean dip would go a long way to keep you blood pressure in check. Eat whole grains such as quinoa or brown rice; and lean proteins such as lean pork, fish or chicken. Avoid foods and drinks that are high in sugar, high in salt as well as high fat snacks.

Servings

It is important to monitor your daily number of servings from various food groups. This number depends on your required amount of calories in a day. For instance, if you want to stick to 2,000 calorie per day, there are specific numbers of servings from various food groups that you can eat. Thankfully, this is outlined below.

Daily Servings permissible on the Dash diet:

- Grains: 7-8 servings. Grains include pasta or rice. Servings may include 1 slice of bread or 1/2 cup of cooked rice.

- Vegetables: 4-5 servings. Go for fiber-rich veggies that are packed with potassium and magnesium. These include dark leafy greens and sweet potatoes. A serving of this, for instance, is one cup of leafy greens.

- Low-Fat Or No-Fat Dairy Foods: 2-3 servings. Go for milk or yogurt and eat cheese sparingly as it has high sodium content. 1 serving may include a cup of yoghurt or milk and one half ounce of cheese.

- Poultry, Meat & Fish: 1-2 servings. Go for lean cuts of red meat, pork and poultry to obtain your daily allowance. The DASH Diet permits a maximum of 6 lean meat servings in a day. However, it is better to avoid it if you can by going for protein-rich veggies like beans and chickpeas.

- Fats And Oils: 2-3 servings. A serving of fat may be 1 tablespoon of oil, 1 teaspoon of margarine or 2 tablespoons of prepared salad dressing.

- Fruits: 4-5 servings. Your best choices are fruits that have high fiber, potassium, and magnesium content, such as pears and apples. Any fruit that can be eaten with the skin on is highly recommended on account of their extra fiber content. A serving is a medium or half cup of fruit (fresh or frozen).

Weekly servings permissible on the dash diet include:

- <u>Nuts, Seeds As Well As Dry Beans</u>: 4-5 servings per week. 1 serving of seeds = 2 tablespoons.

- <u>Sweets</u>: 5 servings or less in a week. Sweets should contain little or no added sugar.

Tips For A Healthy DASH Diet Eating Plan

- Whole grain products are fiber-rich and filling. Choose whole wheat bread or brown rice rather than highly processed white rice or flour products.

- Get 27% of your daily calorie intake from monounsaturated fats. Fat enables the body to absorb minerals and support immune function. Unsalted nuts are great source of monounsaturated fats.

- Calcium is important for bones and for regulating blood pressure. While dairy foods have high calcium content, high-fat dairy also contains saturated fats which are dangerous to heart health. Therefore, ensure you get non-dairy sources of calcium such as soy beans and collard greens as well as beverages like almond milk.

- Read food labels to ensure that the products you use are lower in sodium. Add little or no salt when cooking.

- Include vegetables in your meals. To make it easier for you, always add an extra serving of vegetable to your lunch or dinner. Freeze fresh vegetables to add to soups, stir-fries, sauces and casseroles anytime.

- Add low-fat milk to your meals, including your homemade soups and cooked cereals. Instead of sweetened drinks, take low-fat milk. Take low-fat yoghurt as snack or a piece of low-fat cheese.

- Avoid processed foods.

100 DASH DIET RECIPES

9

BREAKFAST AND SMOOTHIES RECIPES

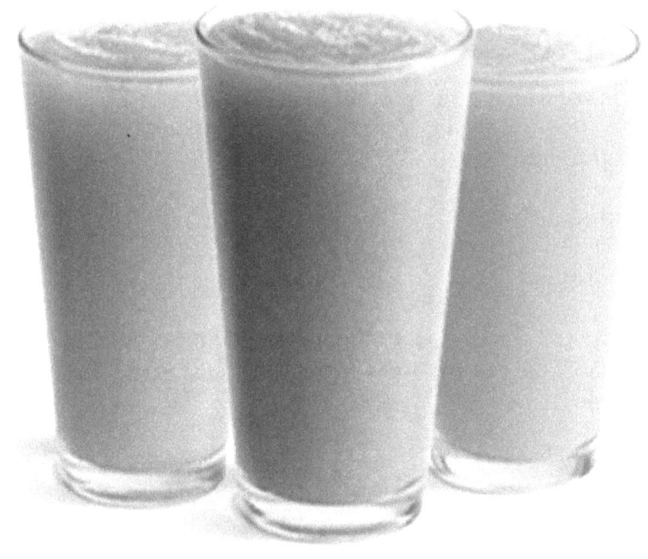

Dash Fruity Smoothie

Preparation time: 10 minutes

Cooking time: 0 min

Servings: 4

Ingredients:

2 oranges, juice

1 cup of pineapple, fresh

1 cup of strawberries, fresh

½ cup of cantaloupe or other melon

1 tbsp honey

1 cup water

Directions:

1. Take out the rind from the melon and pineapple then slice them into chunks. Take out the stems from the strawberries. Refrigerate the fruits to save until later.

2. Once you're ready to serve, transfer all the ingredients into a blender then puree until smooth. Serve chilled.

<u>Note:</u> This can be arranged ahead of time.

Nutritional Information: Calories: 72, Fat: 0g, Cholesterol: 0g, Sodium: 8mg, Carbs: 17g, Protein: 1g

Gumbo Fruitie Smoothie

This refreshing smoothie is packed with vitamins A and C.

Preparation time: 5 minutes

Cooking time: 0 min

Servings: 4

Ingredients:

½ cup of strawberries + ½ cup of blueberries or blackberries

1 banana

4 tbsp of lemon juice (juice of 1 lemon)

1 tbsp of fresh mint to taste

2 cups of fresh raw baby spinach (about 2 oz.)

1 cup cold water/ice

Directions:

1. Pour all the ingredients into a juicer or blender then puree. Enjoy.

Nutritional Information: Calories: 52, Fat: 0g, Cholesterol: 0mg, Sodium: 14mg, Carbs: 12g, Protein: 1g

Creamy Orangy Smoothie

This drink is an amazing source of potassium which aids blood pressure regulation and cell function.

Preparation time: 5 minutes

Cooking time: 0 min

Servings: 2

Ingredients:

¼ of cup orange juice concentrate, frozen

1 cup no-fat vanilla frozen yogurt

¾ cup no-fat milk

Directions:

1. Pour all the ingredients into a blender then blend until smooth.

2. Pour smoothie into chilled-frost tall glasses then serve at once.

Note: You may use a banana instead of the orange juice.

Nutritional Information: Calories: 180, Fat: Cholesterol: 2mg, Sodium: 113mg, Carbs: 0g, Protein: 7g

Creamy Protein Fruity Smoothie

Preparation time: 5 minutes

Cooking time: 0 min

Servings: 1

Ingredients:

1 medium-sized banana, sliced into chunks

1 cup of vanilla yogurt

2 tbsps protein powder

1 cup of 2% milk

2 tbsp wheat germ

Directions:

1. Pour all the ingredients into a blender then blend until smooth.

2. Pour the smoothie into a tall chilled-frost glass then serve at once.

Note: If you want more calories, add 1 tbsp of flaxseed oil to get extra 120 calories, 14g of fat, and no trace of extra cholesterol and sodium.

Nutritional Information: Calories: 608, Fat: 20g, Cholesterol: 57mg, Sodium: 301mg, Carbs: 75, Protein: 32g

Apple-Oat Cinnamon Muffins

Preparation time: 20 minutes

Cooking time: 22 minutes

Servings: 16

Ingredients:

2 medium Granny Smith apples, peeled and chopped

2 ¼ tsp cinnamon

¾ cup milled oats

¼ cup flaxseed meal

1 cup plain Greek yogurt

1 cup all-purpose flour

2 eggs

2 tbsp canola oil

2 tsp vanilla extract

1 ½ tsp baking powder

1 cup + 2 tbsp sugar

½ tsp salt

Directions:

1. Heat oven to 350°F. Oil 2 muffin tins lightly with cooking spray.

2. Mix eggs, yoghurt, vanilla and oil in a mixing bowl. In another medium bowl, mix flour, flaxseed, 1 cup of sugar, oats, baking powder, and two tsp of cinnamon and salt together.
3. Lower the mixer to low speed then add the dry ingredients slowly to the wet ingredients.

4. Mix everything until the batter is just combined and lumpy. Mix in the apples with a spatula then scoop ¼ cup of the batter into each muffin.

5. In a separate small bowl, mix the remaining ¼ tsp of cinnamon and 2 tbsp of sugar together then sprinkle mixture over the batter in each muffin.

6. Bake muffins for about 22 minutes or until the surface turns golden brown and toothpick comes out clean when dipped into the middle.

Note: whole flaxseed and whole oats can be used by milling them in a food processor.

Nutritional Information: Calories: 152, Fat: 2g, Cholesterol: 24mg, Sodium: 122mg, Carbs: 29g, Protein: 4g

Dash Grainy Pancakes

These pancakes are filled with healthy whole grains that help control your appetite.

Preparation time: 40 minutes

Cooking time: 20 minutes

Servings: 18

Ingredients:

1 cup whole-wheat flour

3 large egg whites

2 tbsp ground flaxseed

½ cup of barley flour

¼ cup of millet flour

1 ½ tbsp baking powder

¼ cup rolled oats

2 ¼ cups soy milk

3 tbsp honey

1 tbsp oil

Directions:

1. Combine all the dry ingredients in a large bowl.

2. In another bowl, mix the wet ingredients together which comprises of egg whites, honey, soy milk, and oil.

3. Pour the wet mixture into the dry ingredients then stir until just combined. Refrigerate the batter for about 30 minutes to rest.

4. Preheat the pan on medium heat then scoop about ¼ cup of the batter into the pan to make 1 pancake.

5. Cook until small bubbles begin to appear and the edges start to look dry. 6. Flip the pancake and cook the second side until brown. Transfer to warmed plates then top with fresh fruit or sprinkle with cinnamon/powdered sugar. Serve.

Nutritional Information: Calories: 90, Fat: 2g, Cholesterol: 0mg, Sodium: 115mg, Carbs: 15g, Protein 3g

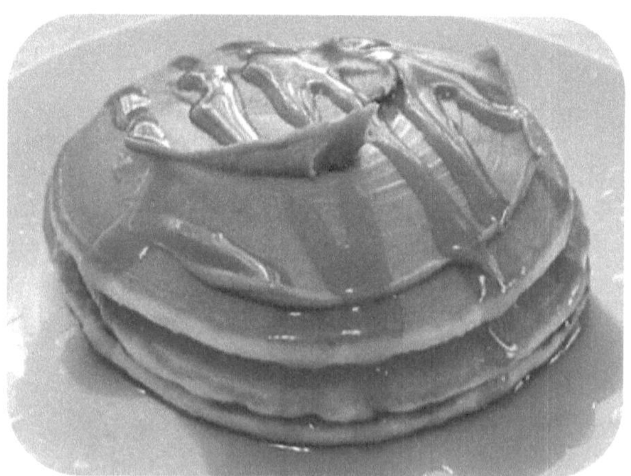

Pancake

Steamy Gumbo Grain Cereal

Make a large dash diet friendly cereal on the weekend then reheat all through the week. Garnish with fruits or yogurt for extra natural sweetness.

Preparation time: 10 minutes

Cooking time: 50 minutes

Servings: 14

Ingredients:

3 tbsp of quinoa, uncooked

½ cup of red wheat berries, uncooked

½ cup pearl barley, uncooked

½ cup of brown rice, uncooked

¼ cup of steel cut oats, uncooked

2 tbsp of flaxseed

6 cups of water

½ tsp kosher salt

Directions:

1. Combine the quinoa, barley, flaxseed, oats, rice, wheat and salt in a large saucepan.

2. Pour in water then stir. Allow it boil over medium heat.
3. Turn down the heat to low then simmer for 45 minutes, stirring from time to time.

Nutritional Information: Calories: 114, Fat: 1g, Cholesterol: 74mg, Sodium: 21mg, Carbs: 3g, Protein 4g

Dash Cinnamon Vanilla Toast

Preparation time: 5 minutes

Cooking time: 10 minutes

Servings: 2

Ingredients:

4 slices cinnamon bread

¼ tsp of ground cinnamon

1 tsp of vanilla

4 egg whites

¼ cup of maple syrup

1/8 tsp ground nutmeg

Directions:

1. Combine nutmeg, vanilla and egg whites in a small bowl. Whisk until it evenly combined.

2. Dip the cinnamon bread into the egg mixture, making sure both sides are well coated.

3. Heat a griddle or nonstick frying pan over medium heat. Once droplet of water sizzles as it touched the pan, add the bread.

4. Sprinkle with ground cinnamon then cook each side for about 4 to 5 minutes or until golden brown.

5. Serve 2 slices of cinnamon toast on warmed individual plates then add 2 tbsp of maple syrup and 1 tsp of powdered sugar to each serving. Serve at once.

Nutritional Information: Calories: 299, Fat: 3g, Cholesterol: 0mg, Sodium: 334mg, Carbs: 57g, Protein 11g

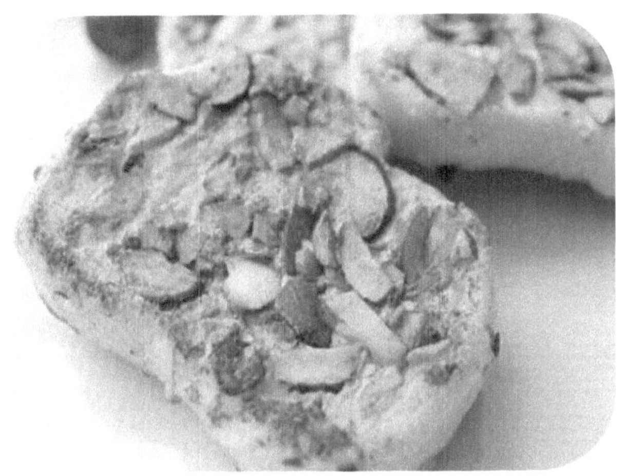

Almond Crusted Toast

Fruity Veggie Blast

Preparation time: 5 minutes

Cooking time: 0 minute

Servings: 1

Ingredients:

½ cup of grapes

½ cup of spinach

½ cup of raspberries

½ cup of kale

½ cup of blueberries

½ beet

½ pear

¼ avocado

1 ½ Cups Water

Directions:

1. In your tall cup, combine all the ingredients then extract for 30 seconds or until smooth. Enjoy!

Nutritional Information: Calories: 301.8, Fat: 8.8 g, Cholesterol: 0.0 mg, Sodium: 64.7 mg, Carbs: 52.5 g, Protein: 4.5 g

Dash Mexican Chicken Bake

Preparation time: 20 minutes

Cooking time: 45 minutes

Servings: 4

Ingredients:

1 lb. chicken breast, skinless, boneless and chopped into bite-sized pieces

1 (15 oz.) can unsalted black beans, drained then rinsed

1 ½ cups of cooked brown rice

2 (14.5 oz.) cans unsalted tomatoes, chopped or mashed

1 cup yellow corn kernels, frozen

1 cup of diced red bell pepper

¼ cup of jalapeno pepper slices (optional)

1 tbsp powdered chili

1 tbsp cumin

1 cup diced poblano pepper

4 cloves of garlic, crushed

1 cup shredded low-fat Monterey Jack cheese

Directions:

1. Preheat the oven to 400°F. Disperse rice in a shallow 3-quart casserole. Place the chicken on top.

2. Combine beans, tomatoes, peppers, corn, garlic and seasoning in a bowl then pour the mixture over the chicken.

3. Top with cheese and jalapeno if you like then bake for 45 minutes.

Nutritional Information: Calories: 325, Fat: 7.1 g, Cholesterol: 57mg, Sodium: 356mg, 6.9 g Carbs: 6.9g, Protein: 28.4 g

Super Morning Bread Pudding
This delicious bread pudding is low in fat and calories.

Preparation time: 24 hours

Cooking time: 1 hour

Servings: 4

Ingredients:

4 slices of whole wheat bread, (about 3 cups cubed)

1 ½ cups of reduced fat milk, or no-fat or 1% fat milk

½ cup of chopped peeled apple

¼ cup raisins

4 eggs

2 tbsp brown sugar

2 tsp powdered sugar (optional)

½ tsp vanilla extract

½ tsp ground cinnamon

1/8 tsp salt

Directions:

1. Preheat the oven to 350°F.

2. Combine eggs, milk, cinnamon, vanilla, brown sugar and salt in a large bowl then whisk until properly mixed.

3. Pour in the chopped apples, bread cubes and raisins then stir until all the ingredients incorporates and the bread cubes are drenched in most of the liquid.

4. Grease an 8" square baking dish with butter or non-stick spray.

5. Pour the mixed bread into the coated baking pan then cover with foil and bake. You may likewise choose to refrigerate for up to 24 hours.

6. Transfer the bread pudding to the oven then bake for 40 minutes. Remove the cover and continue baking for another 20 minutes or until golden brown.

7. Let it sit for 10 minutes before you serve. Sprinkle with powdered sugar if you like.

Nutritional Information: Calories: 250, Fat: 6 g, Sodium: 320 mg, Protein 13 g

Breakfast Applesauce Wheat Toast

Preparation time: 10 minutes

Cooking time: 15 minutes

Servings: 6

Ingredients:

6 whole wheat bread slices

½ cup of milk

2 eggs

¼ cup of applesauce, unsweetened

1 tsp ground cinnamon

2 tbsp white sugar

Directions:

1. Combine milk, eggs, applesauce, cinnamon and sugar in a large mixing bowl and mix properly.

2. Drench each slice of bread in the mixture until well soaked.

3. Coat the skillet or griddle lightly and cook both sides over medium heat until golden brown. Serve immediately.

Nutritional Information: Calories: 150, Fat: 3g, Sodium 220mg, Carbs: 27g, Protein 8g

Deli Berry Oat Muffins

Preparation time: 30 minutes

Cooking time: 20 minutes

Servings: 12

Ingredients:

2/3 cup blueberries, frozen

½ cup raw old-fashioned whole oatmeal

1 ½ cups of flour

½ tsp baking powder

½ cup of dry milk + 1 cup of milk

1/3 cup sugar

1 egg

¼ tsp baking soda

¼ cup oil

½ tsp salt

Directions:

1. Preheat the oven to 350°F. Coat a muffin tin with cooking oil spray.

2. In a bowl, combine the dry ingredients which comprises of flour, baking powder, oatmeal, baking soda, sugar and salt.

3. In a separate bowl, combine the wet ingredients which comprises of egg, dry milk, milk and oil.

4. Pour the wet ingredients into the dry ingredients then mix partially. Now add the blueberries.

5. Stir gently until the batter is lumpy then scoop into the muffin tins.

6. Bake for 20 minutes or until the edges of the muffins are brown. Transfer muffins to a rack then serve warm or cool. Store in an airtight container then refrigerate.

Nutritional Information: Calories: 150, Fat: 5g, Sodium: 180 mg, Carbs: 22g, Protein: 4g, Fiber: 1g

LUNCH RECIPES

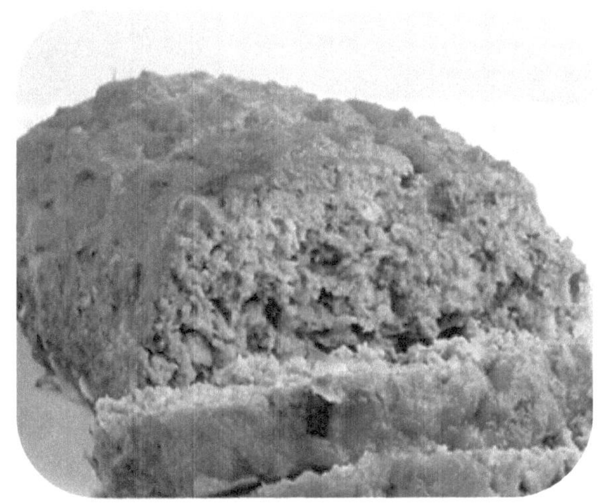

Chili Chick-Lime Tacos

Prepare moist delicious chicken tacos flavored with limes. The perfect healthy lunch at all times.

Preparation time: 10 minutes

Cooking time: 6 hours, 30 minutes

Servings: 6

Ingredients:

1 ½ lbs. chicken breast, halves, boneless and skinless

1 tbsp powdered chili

3 tbsp lime juice

Lime zest

1 cup of chunky salsa

1 cup thawed frozen corn

12 no-fat flour tortillas, warmed (about 6")

Optional ingredients:

Jalapenos, sour cream, shredded lettuce, 2% shredded Mexican cheese

Directions:

1. Set the chicken in a 3-qt. slow cooker. Mix the powdered chili and lime juice together then pour over the chicken.

2. Cover the slow cooker and cook for 5 to 6 hours on low until tender.

3. Take out the chicken. Once it's cool enough to touch, using two forks, shred the meat then return to the slow cooker. Stir in salsa and corn then cook, covered, for about 30 minutes on low setting until well heated.

4. Once done, spoon filling on crispy tacos or tortillas then add preferred optional ingredients like jalapenos, sour cream, cheese and lettuce.

Nutritional Information: Calories: 291, Fat 3g, Cholesterol: 63mg, Sodium: 674mg, Carbs: 37g, Protein 28g

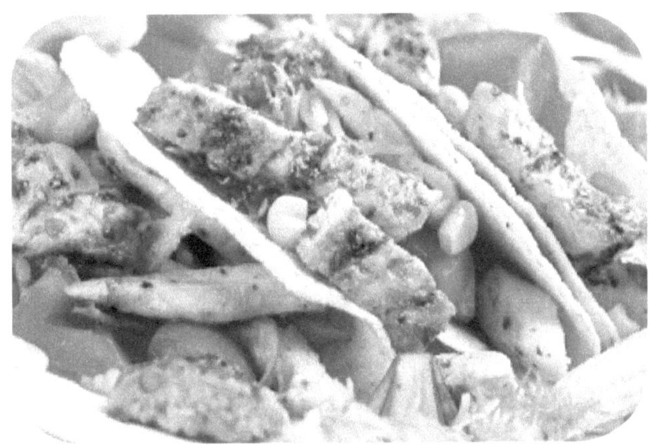

Dash Veggie Balsamic Chicken

Preparation time: 10 minutes

Cooking time: 13 minutes

Servings: 4

Ingredients:

1 ¼ pounds chicken breast tenderloins

3 tbsp balsamic vinegar

¼ cup + 2 tbsp Italian salad dressing

1 cup grape tomatoes, halved

1 ½ cups matchstick carrots

1 pound fresh asparagus, cut off tough ends then dice into 2" pieces (or green beans)

1 ½ tbsp of honey

1/8 tsp crushed red pepper flakes

2 tbsp olive oil

Black pepper, freshly ground

Salt

Directions:

1. Whisk the balsamic vinegar, salad dressing, pepper flakes and honey together in a mixing bowl then set it aside.

2. In a 12" skillet, heat up olive oil over medium-high heat.

3. Season the chicken with pepper and salt to taste and then set the chicken in the skillet. 4. Cook about 6 to 7 minutes, turning once its halfway through cooking time, do this until the chicken is properly cooked. While the chicken is cooking, dice the tomatoes and asparagus.

5. Add half the dressing mixture to the skillet the turn the chicken to evenly coat.

6. Transfer the chicken to a serving platter or large plate but leave the sauce in the skillet.

7. Pour the chopped tomatoes and asparagus into the skillet then season with pepper and salt to taste.

8. Cook for about 4 minutes, stirring consistently until it becomes crisp tender.

9. Transfer the cooked veggies to the platter or plate with chicken.

10. Pour the rest of the dressing mixture into the skillet and cook for about 1 minute, stirring frequently until it becomes thick.

11. Add tomatoes to veggies and chicken then drizzle the dressing mixture on top. You may likewise return the veggies and chicken to the pan and toss until well coated.

Nutritional Information: Calories: 342, Fat: 14g, Cholesterol: 90mg, Sodium: 351mg, Carbs: 20g, Protein 33g

Spicy Avocado Shrimpy Slaw With Lettuce

Preparation time: 15 minutes

Cooking time: 10 minutes

Servings: 1

Ingredients:

For lettuce wraps:

2 big romaine lettuce leaves, Cut off the top and use that, throw away the light green, crunchy bottom

For the shrimp:

6 large shrimps, peeled and deveined

1/8 tsp of cayenne pepper

½ tsp of powdered chili

½ tsp of paprika

½ tsp of cumin

½ tsp of powdered garlic

1 tsp of olive oil

¼ tsp salt

For the slaw:

¾ cup of shredded cole slaw mix

1/3 tsp of honey

2 tsps fresh lime juice

2 tsp of diced cilantro

other ingredients:

1 jalapeno, sliced very thinly (optional)

½ avocado, sliced thinly

Cilantro, diced (optional)

Directions:

1. First, put together the slaw so that the flavors can blend together while you do other things.

2. In a bowl, combine the shredded cole slaw mix, honey, cilantro and lime juice then stir properly until everything mixes together completely. Season with pepper and salt to taste then set it aside

3. In a small bowl, combine chili powder, powdered garlic, cumin, cayenne pepper, paprika and salt. Place the shrimp a plate then season both sides generously with the seasoning mix

4. Heat up 1 tsp of olive oil in a skillet over medium-high heat.

5. Once hot, add the seasoned shrimp then sear both sides until well cooked.

6. To arrange; spoon half the slaw on each romaine leaf then add half of the avocado slices, few jalapenos, three shrimps and then sprinkle cilantro on top

Nutritional Information: Calories: 256, Fat: 18g, Cholesterol: 116 mg, Sodium: 165 mg, Carb: 16g, Protein: 14g

Cheesy Potato Beef Pie

Preparation time: 15 minutes

Cooking time: 50 minutes

Servings: 6

Ingredients:

1 lb. lean ground beef

2 large baking potatoes, peeled and chopped

4 cups of mixed veggies, frozen

½ cup of reduced-fat milk

1 medium onion, diced

½ cup of shredded cheddar cheese

1 garlic clove, crushed

2 tbsp of flour

¾ cup of low sodium beef broth

Ground pepper, to taste

Directions:

1. Pour chopped potatoes into a saucepan, pour in enough water to cover a bit then bring to boil. Lower the heat then simmer for about 15 minutes or until soft while the pan is covered.

2. Drain the potatoes then mash them. Pour in milk then set the mixture aside.

3. Preheat the oven to 375°F.

4. In a large skillet, brown the meat, garlic and onion then stir in flour. Cook for a minute, stirring frequently.

5. Add the veggies and pour in the broth. Cook for 5 minutes until it becomes bubbly then stir properly.

6. Scoop the veggie mixture into a 8" square baking dish then spread the potato mixture on top. Sprinkle with cheese then bake for 25 minutes, until hot and bubbly.

Nutritional Information: Calories: 320, Fat: 7g, Sodium 200 mg, Carbs: 39 g, Protein: 24 g

Smoky Cheese Chicken Quesadillas

Preparation time: 30 minutes

Cooking time: 15 minutes

Servings: 6

Ingredients:

½ cup hot or smoky salsa

4 (4 oz. each) chicken breasts, boneless and skinless

1 cup of shredded low-fat cheddar cheese

1 cup diced fresh tomatoes

1 cup diced onions

6 whole-wheat 8" tortillas

1 cup of diced fresh cilantro

Directions:

1. Heat up oven to 425°F. Coat the baking sheet lightly with cooking spray.

2. Chop the chicken breasts into cubes.

3. Heat up a large, nonstick frying pan then add the cubed chicken and onions then sauté for about 5 to 7 minutes or until the chicken is properly cooked and the onions are tender.

4. Take out from heat then stir in the tomatoes, salsa and cilantro.

5. To put them together; spread a tortilla flat then rub water on the outside edge.

6. Now spread about ½ cup of the chicken mixture on the tortilla, sparing about ½ inch free around the outer edges.

7. Sprinkle a spoonful of shredded cheese on top then fold the tortilla in half then seal.

8. Place the filled tortilla on a cookie sheet then repeat assembling process with the rest of the filling and tortillas.

9. Coat the surface of the tortillas lightly with cooking spray then bake or ablout 5 to 7 minutes until the quesadillas are a bit browned and crispy.

10. Slice in half then serve at once.

Nutritional Information: Calories: 298; Fat: 5g; Cholesterol 70mg; Sodium 524mg; Carbs 25g; Protein 27g

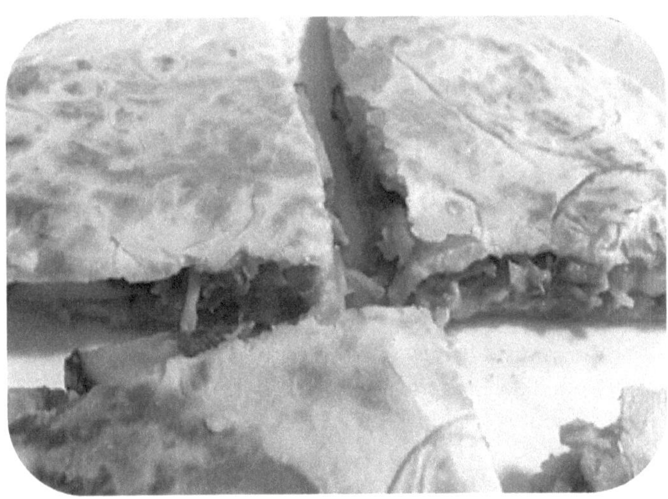

Cheesy Tuna Muffin Melts

Preparation time: 10 minutes

Cooking time: 5 minutes

Servings: 4

Ingredients:

3 oz. low-fat Cheddar cheese, grated

6 oz. white tuna packed in water, drained

2 whole-wheat English muffins, halved

1/3 cup of diced celery

¼ cup reduced-fat salad dressing

¼ cup of diced onion

Black pepper and salt to taste

Directions:

1. Preheat the broiler.

2. Mix the drained tuna, salad dressing, onion and celery then season with pepper and salt.

3. Toast the muffin halves then place the split side facing upwards on the baking sheet. Top each muffin halves with ¼ of the tuna mixture then broil for 2 to 3 minutes or until well heated.

4. Add cheese on top then return to the broiler and broil for another 1 minute until the cheese completely melts.

Nutritional Information: Calories: 210; Fat: 6 g; Carbs: 20 g; Sodium 417mg; Protein: 19g;

Tuna Spinach Dill Sandwiches

Preparation time: 20 minute

Cooking time: 0 minute

Servings: 4

Ingredients:

8 slices of whole wheat sandwich bread

1 (6.4 oz.) light tuna packed in water

1 cup fresh baby spinach

½ tsp dill weed

½ medium cucumber, peeled, deseeded then chopped

Juice of 1 lemon

¼ cup peeled chopped red onion (about ½ small one)

2 ribs celery, chopped

2 tbsp olive oil

¼ tsp freshly ground black pepper

½ tsp unsalted seasoning blend

Directions:

1. Mix the tuna, dill weed, celery, onion and cucumber together.

2. Sprinkle lemon juice and olive oil on top then stir. Season with pepper and seasoning blend.

3. Assemble the sandwich with ¼ cup of baby spinach leaves and ½ cup of tuna salad. Press the spinach and tuna down to compact.

Note: This recipe will make 2 cups of tuna that should be refrigerated for up to 3 days or longer for more meals.

Nutritional information: Calories: 194, Fat: 3g; Cholesterol: 14 mg, Sodium: 450mg; Carb: 27 g; Protein: 17 g

Dash Veggie Hummus Wrap

Preparation time: 12 minutes

Cooking time: 0 minute

Servings: 1

Ingredients:

1/3 cup of hummus

8 fresh mint leaves

1 cup baby lettuce mix

¼ whole long English cucumber

1 (8") whole-wheat tortillas

1 plum tomato

1 tsp of lemon juice

¼ medium red onion

½ tsp of lemon zest

½ tsp of ground black pepper

Directions:

1. Disperse the hummus on the tortilla then place the rest of the ingredients on top.

2. Tightly roll up the tortilla. Enjoy!

Note: You can substitute other healthy veggies for the ones used in this recipe. You can also use any preferred flavored hummus.

Nutrition information: Calories: 319, Fat: 12g, Cholesterol: 0mg, Sodium: 557mg, Carb: 40g, Protein: 13g

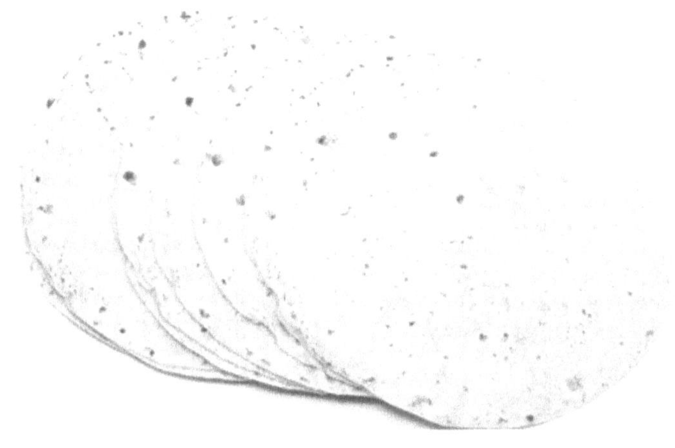

Tortillas

Hot Tomato Bean Chili

Preparation time: 15 minutes

Cooking time: 20 minutes

Servings: 4

Ingredients:

30 oz reduced-sodium red kidney beans

1 jalapeno pepper

1 cup of canned crushed tomatoes

1 ½ tsp of powdered chili

2 tsp of grapeseed oil

1 medium red onion

2 garlic clove

1 ¼ cups reduced-sodium veggie broth

½ tsp of sea salt

Directions:

1. In a large saucepan, heat up oil over medium-high. Add the jalapeno and onion then sauté for about 5 minutes until the onion is a bit caramelized. Add the garlic then sauté for about 30 seconds until aromatic.

2. Stir in the rest of the ingredients then bring to boil for a minute on high heat.

3. Cover and lower heat to low. Simmer for about 10 minutes until the flavors incorporate. Simmer uncovered over medium-low heat for a thick consistency.

4. Top with reduced fat cream and fresh cilantro if desired.

Nutrition Information: Calories: 270; Fat: 2g; Cholesterol: 0mg; Sodium: 643mg; Carbs: 45g; Protein: 17g

Veggie Chicken Rotisserie Salad With Bean Tarragon Dressing

Preparation time: 20 minutes

Cooking time: 0 minute

Servings: 4

Ingredients:

1 1/3 cups of cooked chicken breast

15 ounce canned white beans

1 tbsp extra-virgin olive oil

1/3 cup of white balsamic vinegar

2 garlic cloves

6 cups salad mix

2 tbsp fresh tarragon

½ medium red onion

12 red/green grapes

1 cup of English cucumber

¾ tsp of ground black pepper

3 tbsp of pine nuts

Directions:

1. In a blender, combine ½ cup of the beans, 1 tbsp of tarragon, garlic, oil and vinegar. Cover then puree.

2. Assemble the greens on a large platter then top with chicken, the remaining beans, 1 tbsp of tarragon, cucumber, pepper, onion, grapes and nuts.

3. Serve with dressing on the side.

Nutrition information: Calories: 357; Fat: 11g; Cholesterol: 0mg; Sodium: 65mg; Carbs: 39g; Protein: 26g

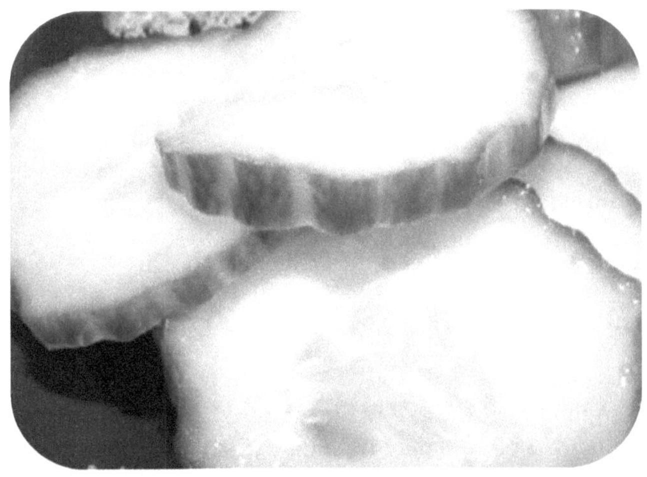

Cucumber

Spinach Oat Nut Stuffed Turkey Burger

Enjoy the goodness of turkey burger stuffed with delicious goodness of spinach, oatmeal and nutmeg. Enjoy!

Preparation time: 20 minutes

Cooking time: 20 minutes

Servings: 4

Ingredients:

12 oz 93% lean ground turkey

1/3 cup of old fashioned rolled oats

3 cups of fresh baby spinach

1 pinch ground nutmeg

1 garlic clove

2 tsp lemon juice

1 egg

½ tsp sea salt

¾ tsp ground black pepper

Directions:

1. Combine all the ingredients in a medium bowl.

2. Coat a large nonstick skillet with cooking spray then set over medium heat.

3. Form the mixture into 4 patties about 5" wide then cook each side in the skillet for about 7 to 8 minutes until well cooked and browned. Serve.

Nutrition information: Calories: 172; Fat: 8g; Cholesterol: 95mg; Sodium: 296mg; Carbs: 6g; Protein 20g

Grilled Gumbo Veggie Sandwich

Preparation time: 5 minutes

Cooking time: 7 minutes

Servings: 1

Ingredients:

2 slices of focaccia bread

Baby spinach

1 small onion, sliced

½ yellow squash, sliced

1 ½ tbsp mayonnaise

½ cup sliced red bell pepper

¼ cup crumbled no-fat cheese

2 tbsp olive oil

1 garlic clove

½ zucchini, sliced

½ tbsp lemon juice

Directions:

1. In a bowl, combine mayonnaise, garlic and lemon juice then refrigerate.

2. Preheat the grill over high heat then coat the veggies with olive oil. Coat the grill rack.

3. Grill all the veggies for 3 to 5 minutes. Note that the peppers might take a bit longer. Remove the veggies from the grill then set aside.

4. Spread the mayonnaise evenly on the bread slices then sprinkle feta cheese on top.

5. Place on the grill with the cheese side facing up. Cover with lid for 2 minutes then remove bread from the grill and then top with the veggies.

6. Serve open grilled sandwich. .

Note: Serve with berries and reduced-fat yoghurt for a more dash friendly meal.

Nutritional Information: Calories: 240, Fat: 14 g, Sodium: 490 mg, Carb: 24 g, Protein: 7 g,

Dash Tomato Beef Cabbage

Preparation time: 10 minutes

Cooking time: 40 minutes

Servings: 6

Ingredients:

1 tbsp oil

1 - 2 lbs. lean ground beef

1 large onion, diced

1 garlic clove, minced

1 small cabbage, diced

1 (8 oz.) canned tomato sauce

2 (14.5 oz each) cans of chopped tomatoes

½ cup of water

Cinnamon, cayenne pepper and paprika, to taste

1 tsp ground black pepper

1 tsp sea salt

Directions:

1. Heat up olive oil in a large skillet over medium heat. Add onion and the ground beef then cook, stirring, until the onion is soft and the beef is no longer pink.

2. Add the garlic then continue cooking for a minute.

3. Add the diced cabbage, tomato sauce, pepper, tomatoes and salt, and bring to boil. Cover then simmer for 20 to 30 minutes until the cabbage is soft.

Nutritional Information: Calories: 283.3; Fat: 18.4 g; Cholesterol: 56.7 mg; Sodium: 757.0 mg; Carbs: 14.3 g; Protein: 16.5 g

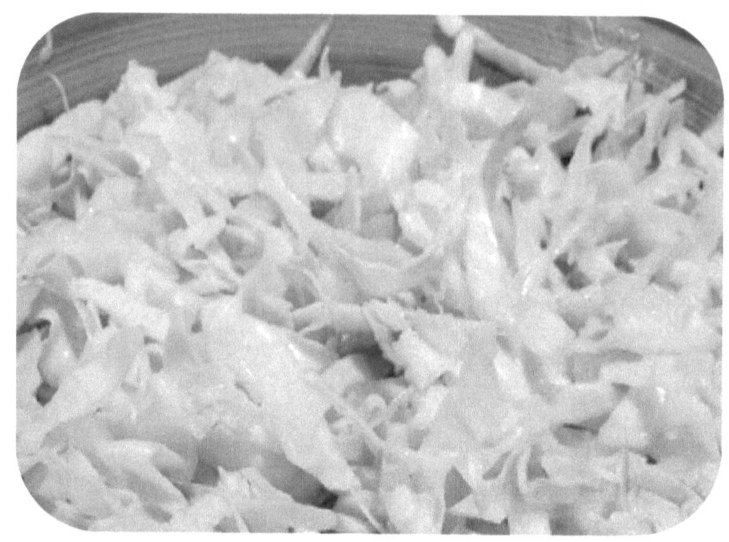

Diced Cabbage

DINNER RECIPES

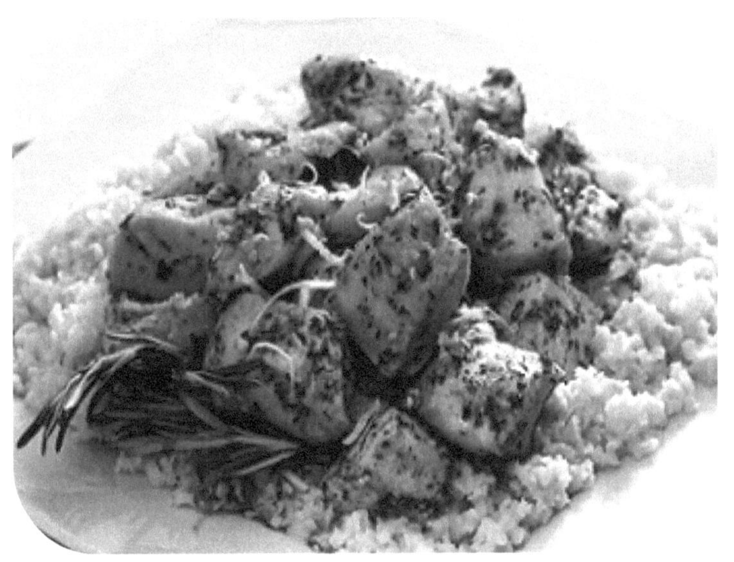

Cheesy Chicken Spinach Tortilla Casserole

Preparation time: 45 minutes

Cooking time: 30 minutes

Servings: 9

Ingredients:

1 lb chicken breasts, boneless, skinless and trimmed

1/3 cup of Mexican cheese blend, shredded

4 oz. goat cheese

2 tbsp extra-virgin olive oil

8 oz. mushroom slices

4 cups of baby spinach

2 cups of reduced-fat milk

1 medium leek, white and light green part, halved then sliced

3 garlic cloves, sliced

1 tbsp of cornstarch

¼ tsp ground pepper

¼ cup diced pickled jalapeños

1/3 cup of green salsa

12 corn tortillas, halved

¼ tsp of salt

Directions:

1. Preheat oven to 400°F. Spray a 9 by 13" baking dish with cooking spray.

2. Set the chicken in a medium saucepan or skillet then add enough water to cover the chicken by 1". Bring to boil, cover then lower heat to low and

gently simmer for 10 to 12 minutes or until the chicken is well cooked and isn't pink in the center.

3. Once cooked, transfer the chicken to a clean cutting board then with two forks, shred or chop.

4. While chopping the chicken, heat up oil in a large pot over medium-high heat. Add the leek, mushrooms and garlic then cook for about 4 minutes, stirring from time to time, until the leek is tender and begins to brown.

5. In a small bowl, whisk milk and cornstarch together then pour into the pot. Cook for 3.5 minutes, stirring regularly until the mixture thickens.

6. Stir in the jalapenos, spinach, pepper, goat cheese and salt, and cook for about 2 extra minutes or until the spinach wilts and the cheese melts.

7. Take out from heat then stir in the chicken.

8. Cover the base of the baking dish with 6 tortilla halves then spread 1½ cups of the filling over the tortillas. Repeat this process with 3 extra layers of tortillas and 2 additional layers of filling, finishing with a layer of tortillas.

9. Spread salsa on top then sprinkle with shredded cheese.

10. Bake for 20 to 25 minutes until hot and bubbly. Allow it sit for up to 10 minutes before serving.

Nutritional Information: Calories: 255; Fat: 10 g; Carbs: 22 g, Protein 20 g; Sodium 281mg; Cholesterol: 49mg

Cilantro Chickpea Curry

Preparation time: 5 minutes

Cooking time: 15 minutes

Servings: 6

Ingredients:

2 (15 oz.) cans chickpeas, rinsed

4 large garlic cloves

1 medium serrano pepper, sliced into thirds

1 medium yellow onion, diced into 1"

1 (2") fresh ginger, peeled then roughly diced

2 tsp ground coriander

6 tbsp grapeseed/canola oil

2 tsp ground cumin

2¼ cups unsalted chopped tomatoes + their juice (28 oz. can)

½ tsp ground turmeric

2 tsp garam masala

¾ tsp kosher salt

For garnish: fresh cilantro

Directions:

1. In a blender, pulse the ginger, garlic and Serrano until crushed. Scrape down the sides then puree again. Add the onion then pulse until much chopped, but not watery.

2. Heat up oil in a large saucepan over medium-high heat. Pour in the onion mixture then cook for 3 to 5 minutes, stirring from time to time until softened. Add the turmeric, cumin and coriander then cook for 2 minutes while stirring.

3. In a blender, pulse the tomatoes until much chopped. Pour tomato puree into the pan; add salt then lower heat to keep up a simmer. Cook for 4 minutes, stirring from time to time.

4. Add the chickpeas and garam masala then lower heat to a low simmer. Cover and cook for 5 more minutes, stirring from time to time. Serve curry garnished with cilantro, if you like.

Nutritional Information: Calories: 278, Fat: 15 g, Cholesterol: 0 mg, Sodium: 354 mg , Carbs: 30 g, Protein: 6 g

Chicken Cauli-Scallion Fried Rice

Preparation time: 30 minutes

Cooking time: 7 minutes

Servings: 4

Ingredients:

4 cups cauliflower rice

3 scallions, separate white and green parts, sliced thinly

1 lb. chicken thighs, boneless, skinless, trimmed then sliced into ½" sizes

1 tsp + 2 tbsp peanut oil, divided

2 large eggs, whisked

1 tsp sesame oil (optional)

½ cup chopped red bell pepper

1 tbsp grated fresh ginger

3 tbsp low-sodium soy sauce or tamari

1 tbsp minced garlic

1 cup of snow peas, trimmed then halved

Directions:

1. In your food processor, pulse cauliflower florets into rice-size granules. Note that 1 (2 lb.) head of cauliflower will give you 4 cups of cauli rice. You may use prepared cauliflower rice.

2. In a large heavy skillet or flat-bottomed carbon-steel wok, heat up one tsp of oil over high heat.

3. Pour in the whisked eggs then fully cook one side for 30 seconds, without stirring, and then flip over and cook for about 15 seconds. Transfer cooked egg to a cutting board then slice into ½" pieces.

4. Pour 1 tbsp of oil into the pan and also the white scallion, garlic and ginger and then cook for about 30 seconds, stirring, until the scallions are soft. Add the chicken then cook for 1 minute while stirring.

5. Add the snow peas and bell pepper and cook, stirring for 2 to 4 minutes until just soft. Transfer everything to a large platter.

6. Pour the remaining one tbsp of oil into the pan; add the cauliflower rice, stirring for about 2 minutes until it starts to soften.

7. Pour the eggs and chicken mixture into the pan. Add soysauce/tamari and sesame oil if you like and then stir until well mixed. Top with scallion greens. Serve.

Note: People who are gluten-sensitive or has celiac disease should use gluten-free soy sauces because soy sauce may contain wheat, sweeteners and flavors.

Nutritional Information: Calories: 304, Fat: 15 g, Cholesterol: 200 mg, Sodium: 591 mg, Carbs: 12 g, Protein: 30 g,

Roasted Garlicky Brussels Salmon

Preparation time: 20 minutes

Cooking time: 25 minutes

Servings: 6

Ingredients:

2 lb. salmon fillet, wild-caught, skinned then sliced into 6 pieces

4 large garlic cloves, divided

6 cups Brussels sprouts, trimmed then sliced

¼ cup extra-virgin olive oil

2 tbsp finely diced fresh oregano, divided

¾ cup white wine

¾ tsp freshly ground pepper, divided

1 tsp salt, divided

Lemon wedges

Directions:

1. Preheat the oven to 450°F.

2. In a small bowl, mince 2 garlic cloves with oil, ¼ tsp of pepper, 1 tbsp of oregano and ½ teaspoon of salt. Slice the remaining garlic in half; in a large roasting pan, toss the garlic with 3 tbsp of seasoned oil and Brussels. Roast for 15 minutes, stirring once.

3. Pour the wine into the remaining oil mixture then take out the pan from the oven. Stir the veggies then set the salmon on top.

4. Pour in the wine mixture slowly then sprinkle with ½ tsp of pepper, the rest of the oregano and ½ tsp of salt.

5. Bake for 5 to 10 minutes until the salmon is cooked through then serve with lemon wedges.

Nutritional Information: Calories: 334, Fat: 15 g, Cholesterol: 71 mg, Sodium: 485 mg , Carbs: 10 g, Protein: 33 g,

Curry Pork Veggie Noodles

Preparation time: 5 minutes

Cooking time: 10 minutes

Servings: 4

Ingredients:

8 oz. rice noodles

8 oz. cooked boneless pork loin/pork tenderloin, chopped into cubes

3 tbsp toasted sesame oil

2 tbsp curry paste, Thai

2 scallions, diced

1 tbsp finely chopped garlic

2 tsp finely chopped fresh ginger

2 tbsp low-sodium soy sauce

1 cup shredded red cabbage

3 tbsp diced fresh cilantro

1 cup diced green beans

1 tsp brown sugar

Directions:

1. Cook the rice noodles according to instructions on the package. Drain, rinse then transfer to a large bowl.

2. In a small saucepan, mix sesame oil, ginger, garlic, scallions and brown sugar. Heat up the mixture over medium heat until it begins to sizzle then cook for 15 seconds.

3. Remove from heat then stir in curry paste and soy sauce. Add the noodles, green beans, pork, cilantro and cabbage then toss gently to combine.

Cooking tip: The noodle mixture and sauce should be refrigerated separately for up to a day then toss them together before you serve.

Note: People who are gluten-sensitive or has celiac disease should use gluten-free soy sauces because soy sauce may contain wheat, sweeteners and flavors.

Nutritional Information: Calories: 407; Fat: 12 g; Cholesterol: 41 mg; Sodium: 487 mg Carbs: 57 g; Protein: 16 g;

Cheesy Veggie Lasagna

This low carb meal is packed with veggies and it's the perfect healthy dinner for the family.

Preparation time: 45 minutes

Cooking time: 45 minutes

Serving: 8

Ingredients:

12 oz. sweet Italian sausage, remove casings

1 large eggplant, sliced lengthwise into ¼" long strips

1 (28 oz.) canned unsalted crushed tomatoes

1 large zucchini, sliced lengthwise into ¼" long strips

½ onion, diced

2 garlic cloves, minced

1 tsp dried basil

¼ cup of dry red wine

1 tsp of dried oregano

1 large egg

1 cup of shredded mozzarella, divided

1 cup ricotta cheese, part-skim

¼ tsp ground pepper

For garnish: fresh basil

Directions:

1. Preheat the oven to 400°F. Oil 2 large baking sheets with cooking spray.

2. Assemble the zucchini and eggplant on the greased baking sheets in a single layer then roast for 20 minutes until soft.

3. On the other hand, cook the sausage in a large saucepan for about 6 minutes until browned, crumbling with a spoon.

4. Add garlic and onion then cook for 2 to 3 minutes, stirring from time to time until soft and aromatic.

5. Pour in the wine, tomatoes, oregano and basil then cook, stirring from time to time until it becomes bubbling. Reduce heat then simmer for 10 minutes.

6. In a small bowl, combine egg, ricotta and pepper.

7. Spread out 1 cup of sauce in a 9 by 13" baking dish then layer with half of the eggplant, glop on 1/3 cup of ricotta mixture then sprinkle ¼ cup of mozzarella on top. 8. Layer half of the zucchini crosswise to the eggplant layer, then top with 1 cup of sauce, glop on 1/3 cup of ricotta mixture then sprinkle ¼ cup of mozzarella on top.

9. Layer the rest of the eggplant then top with 1 cup of sauce, dollop the rest of the ricotta mixture then sprinkle ¼ cup of mozzarella on top. Layer the rest of the zucchini then top with the rest of the sauce and mozzarella.

10. Bake lasagna for about 30 minutes until the sauce becomes bubbling around the rim. Let it sit for 10 to 20 minutes before you serve. Top with fresh basil, if you like.

Nutritional Information: Calories: 279; Fat: 16 g; Carbs: 19 g; Protein: 17 g; Cholesterol: 69 mg; Sodium: 506 mg;

One-Pan Veggie Roasted Chicken

Enjoy a healthy dinner of roasted chicken with deliciously seasoned veggies. Yummy!
Preparation time: 5 minutes

Cooking time: 15 minutes

Servings 2

Ingredients:

2 medium chicken breasts, diced

1 cup of broccoli florets

1 cup of bell pepper, diced

1 zucchini, diced

½ onion, diced

½ cup of tomatoes, diced (or grape/plum)

¼ tsp of paprika (optional)

2 tbsp of olive oil

½ tsp of black pepper

1 tsp Italian seasoning

½ tsp salt

Directions:

1. Preheat the oven to 500°F.

2. Dice all the vegetables into chunky pieces. Chop the chicken into cubes on a separate cutting board.

3. Transfer the cubed chicken and veggies to a medium-sized sheet pan/roasting dish then add olive oil, paprika, Italian seasoning, pepper and salt, and then toss to combine.

4. Bake for about 15 minutes until the chicken is cooked and the vegetables are charred. Serve with pasta, salad or rice. Enjoy.

Nutritional Information: Calories: 241, Fat: 15.2 g, Cholesterol: 55.7mg, Sodium: 357mg, Carbs: 6.g, Protein 19.9g

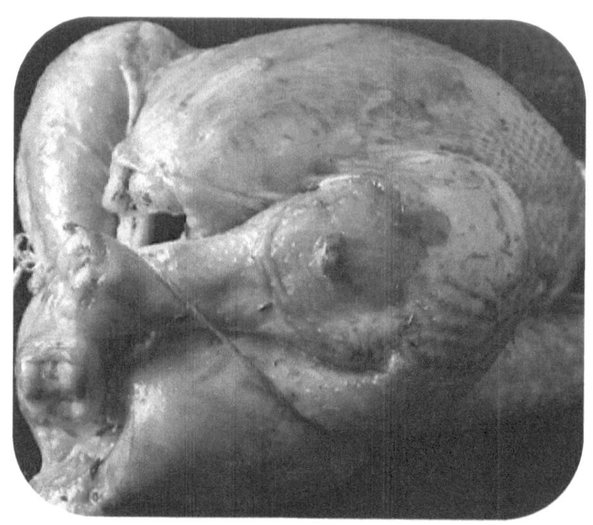

Creamy Crumbly And Whole Wheat Macaroni

Preparation time: 10 minutes

Cooking time: 30 minutes

Servings: 8

Ingredients:

2 cups panko breadcrumbs

¾ lb. whole wheat elbow macaroni

1/3 cup shredded low-fat Cheddar Cheese

1 tsp no-salt added butter

1 ½ cups shredded low-fat Cheddar Cheese

2 ¾ cups of no-fat milk

1 tbsp fresh thyme

2 tsp no-salt added butter

3 tbsp all-purpose flour

1 cup reduced-sodium chicken stock

2 tsp Dijon mustard

1 tbsp fresh thyme

¼ tsp freshly ground black pepper

Directions:

1. Preheat the oven to 400°F. Grease a 3-qt shallow baking dish. Fill a large pot with water about ¾ full then add a pinch of salt. Add the macaroni and cook until al dente.

2. In a sauté pan, melt butter then add panko breadcrumbs. Add pepper and continue stirring over medium heat until it turns golden brown. Allow it cool then add 1/3 cup of Cheddar until mixed.

3. Melt butter in a large saucepan over low to medium heat then stir in flour for 3 minutes. Stir in milk then bring sauce to boil, whisking frequently and simmer.

4. Whisk from time to time for 3 minutes then stir in the remaining 1 ½ cups of Cheddar, thyme, mustard and pepper. Remove pan from heat.

5. In a large bowl, stir the macaroni, sauce and chicken stock together then transfer to the baking dish.

6. Sprinkle cheese mixture and breadcrumbs on top then bake in the center of the oven for 20 to 25 minutes, or until it become bubbling and golden.

Nutritional Information: Calories: 350; Fat: 8g; Carbs: 54g; Protein: 19g; Sodium: 360 mg

Creamy Avocado Lime Tilapia Tacos

Preparation time: 10 minutes

Cooking time: 20 minutes

Preparation: 4

Ingredients:

8 (5") white corn tortillas

1 lb. tilapia filets, rinsed then pat dry

4 tbsp of no-fat sour cream (optional)

8 slices of avocado (1 medium avocado)

1 small onion, diced

2 cups chopped tomatoes

4 garlic cloves, finely chopped

2 jalapeno peppers, deseeded and diced

1 tsp of olive oil

¼ cup of chopped fresh cilantro

3 tbsp lime juice

Pepper and salt to taste

1 cup of shredded cabbage

For garnish: freshly chopped cilantro and lime wedges

Directions:

1. Heat up olive oil in a skillet then sauté onion until transparent. Add garlic and stir well.

2. Place the tilapia in the skillet then cook until the flesh begins to flake.

3. Add tomatoes, lime juice, cilantro and jalapeno peppers then sauté for about 5 minutes over medium-high heat. Break up the fish to get everything combined then season with pepper and salt to taste.

4. On the other hand, heat up each side of tortillas on a skillet for some minutes to warm up.

5. Scoop a bit over ¼ cup of fish mixture on each warmed tortilla then add 2 avocado slices.

6. Share 1 tbsp of sour cream and ¼ cup of shredded cabbage between both tacos.

7. Top with lime wedges and chopped cilantro.

Nutritional Information: Calories: 427; Fat: 12 g; Carbs: 45 g; Protein: 35 g; Sodium: 142 mg

Creamy Mushroom Beef Stroganoff

Preparation time: 10 minutes

Cooking time: 30 minutes

Servings: 4

Ingredients:

½ lb. beef round steak, boneless, fat removed then sliced into ¾" thick

½ cup of diced onion

½ can no-fat cream of mushroom soup, undiluted

4 cups of yolkless egg noodles, uncooked

1 tbsp all-purpose flour

½ tsp of paprika

½ cup of no-fat sour cream

½ cup of water

Directions:

1. Sauté onions for about 5 minutes in a nonstick frying pan over medium heat until they're transparent.

2. Add the beef and keep cooking for extra 5 minutes or until the beef is soft and well browned. Drain properly then set aside.

3. Fill a big pot with water about ¾ full then bring to boil. Add the noodles then cook for 10 to 12 minutes until tender or according to the instructions on the package. Drain the pasta properly.

4. Whisk flour, soup and water together in a saucepan over medium heat then stir for 5 minutes until the sauce becomes thick.

5. Add the paprika and soup mixture to the beef in the frying pan then cook over medium heat. Stir everything together until warmed through.

6. Remove from heat then add the sour cream then stir until well mixed.

7. To serve, share the pasta between the plates then top with the beef mixture and serve at once.

Nutritional Information: Calories: 302; Fat 6g; Protein: 24g; Sodium: 307mg; Carbs: 38g

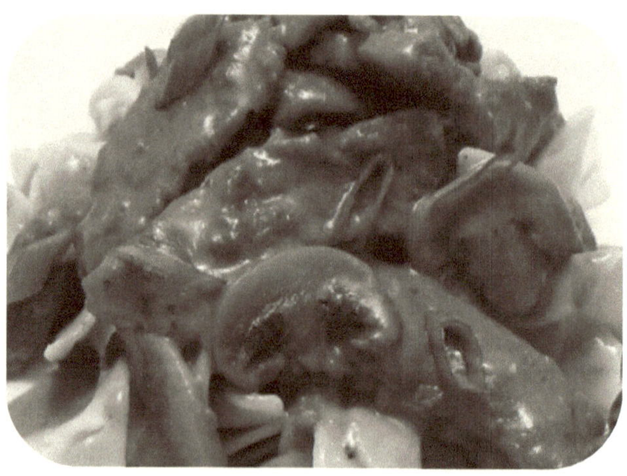

Cheesy Bean Enchiladas

Preparation time: 20 minutes

Cooking time: 20 minutes

Servings: 8

Ingredients:

1 ½ cups low-fat shredded cheese

2 (15 oz.) cans black beans, drained then rinsed

½ cup of salsa

1 (15 oz.) enchilada sauce

8 (10") whole wheat flour tortillas

1 (8 oz) corn, drained

Directions:

1. Preheat the oven to 350°F. Grease a 9 by 13" baking dish lightly.

2. In a bowl, combine half of the cheese, beans, corn and salsa together. Spoon about ½ cup of the bean mixture into each tortilla.

3. Roll up tortilla then place the sealed down on the side in the baking dish. Next pour the enchilada sauce over tortillas then sprinkle the rest of the cheese on top.

4. Bake 15 to 20 minutes or until hot. Refrigerate leftovers within two hours.

Nutritional Information: Calories: 170; Fat: 5 g; Carbs: 23 g; Protein: 8 g; Sodium: 500 mg

Roasted Lemon Salmon

Preparation time: 10 minutes

Cooking time: 22 minutes

Servings: 4

Ingredients:

¼ cup minced fresh dill

4 (6 oz.) wild salmon fillets

1 lemon, sliced into 4 wedges

4 garlic cloves, peeled then finely chopped

Black pepper, freshly ground

Directions:

1. Preheat the oven to 400°F.

2. Oil a glass baking dish with nonstick cooking spray then set the salmon fillets in the baking dish.

3. Squeeze out juice from one lemon wedge over each fillet.

4. Sprinkle salmon with dill, black pepper and garlic.

5. Bake for about 20 to 22 minutes until the center of the salmon is opaque.

Nutritional Information: Calories: 251, Sodium: 78 mg, Fat: 11 g, Cholesterol: 94 mg, Carbs: 2 g, Protein: 34 g

Mayo Celery Chicken Salad

Preparation time: 10 minutes

Cooking time: 30 minutes

Servings: 5

Ingredients:

3 ¼ cups of chicken cubes, skinless and cooked

3 tbsp light mayo whip

¼ cups of chopped celery

½ tsp of powdered onion

1 tbsp lemon juice

Directions:

1. Bake the chicken then slice into cubes, and then refrigerate

2. Mix all the ingredients with chilled chicken together.

Nutritional Information: Calories: 176.5; Fat: 2.7 g; Cholesterol: 88.0 mg; Sodium: 180.0 mg; Carbs: 2.0 g; Protein: 34.2 g

SOUP RECIPES

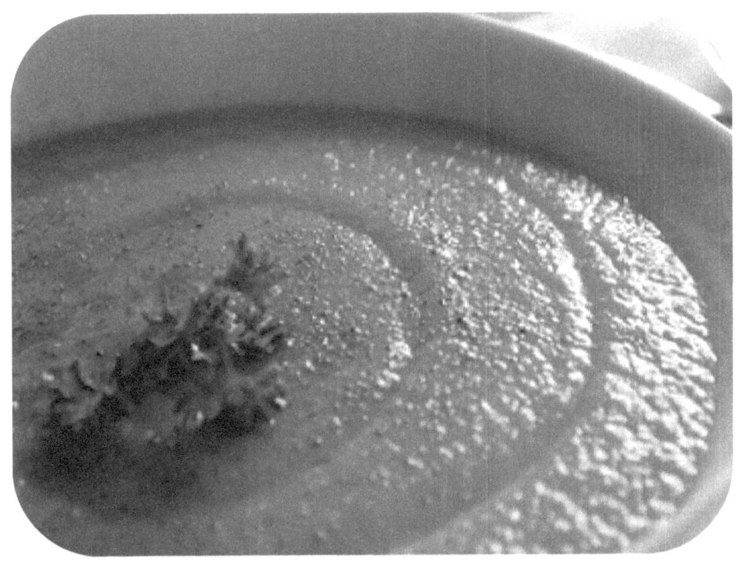

Hot Dash Lentil Stew

This healthy red lentil stew is totally vegan, low in sodium and very nutritious.

Preparation time: 5 minutes

Cooking time: 40 minutes

Servings: 4

Ingredients:

1 cup dried red lentils, rinsed

3 medium peeled carrots, diced

1 yellow onion, diced

1 rib celery, diced

1 small yellow bell pepper, diced

2 garlic cloves garlic, finely chopped

5 cups veggie broth

14 oz. canned reduced-sodium chopped tomatoes

Directions:

1. Spray a large soup pan with veggie oil cooking spray then heat to medium.

2. Add onions and garlic then sauté until translucent.

3. Add the fresh veggies than sauté for 2 to 3 minutes.

4. Pour veggie broth, tomatoes and lentils into the pot then bring to boil.

5. Lower heat to low, cover then simmer for about 30 minutes until the lentils are soft.

6. Scoop stew into soup bowls then serve.

Nutritional Information: Calories: 248; Fat: 1 g; Carbs: 45 g; Protein: 16 g

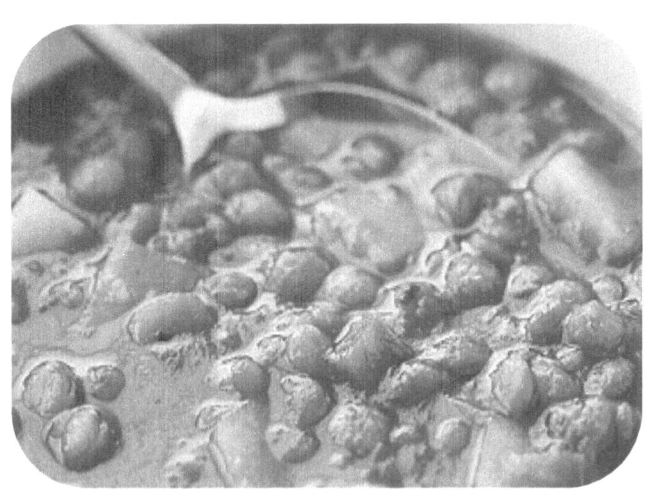

Dash Friendly Veggie Minestrone Soup

Preparation time: 10 minutes

Cooking time: 16 minutes

Servings: 4

Ingredients:

½ cup of diced spinach

1 tbsp olive oil

1/3 cup of diced celery

½ cup diced onion

1 carrot, chopped

4 cups of no-fat, no-salt added chicken broth

1 clove of garlic, finely chopped

½ cup of whole-grain small shell pasta, uncooked

2 large tomatoes, seeded then diced

1 (16 oz.) can chickpeas, drained then rinsed

2 tbsp fresh basil, diced

1 small zucchini, chopped

Directions:

1. Heat up olive oil in a large saucepan over medium heat. Add the celery, onion and carrot then sauté for about 5 minutes until tender.

2. Add the garlic and keep cooking for 1 more minute. Stir in the tomatoes, broth, beans, spinach and pasta then bring to boil over high heat.

3. Lower heat then simmer for 10 minutes. Add the zucchini, cover and cook for 5 more minutes.

4. Remove from heat then stir in basil. Scoop soup into soup bowls then serve at once.

Nutritional Information: Calories: 213; Fat: 5g; Protein: 10g; Carbs: 30g; Sodium 400mg

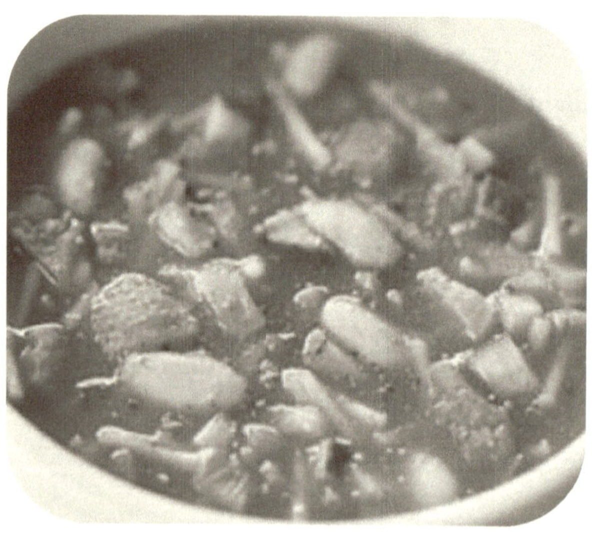

Veggie Sirloin Bean Chili

Preparation time: 20 minutes

Cooking time: 1 hour

Servings: 12

Ingredients:

1 lb ground sirloin, 95% lean

½ bag veggies mix, frozen

½ bag pepper/onion mix, frozen

1 (15 oz) can black beans, drained then rinsed

1 (15 ½ oz) can kidney beans, drained then rinsed

2 - 3 garlic cloves, finely chopped

1 (14 ½ oz) can unsalted chopped tomatoes

1 (15 ½ oz) can unsalted tomato sauce

1 cup of frozen corn

2 tbsp paprika

2 tbsp of powdered chili

Directions:

1. Heat up a big nonstick skillet over medium-high heat. Add the ground beef then cook for 3 to 5 minutes.

2. Add onions, garlic and pepper then cook for 5 minutes over medium heat, until onions becomes soft and translucent. The garlic shouldn't turn brown because it will be bitter.

3. Add the beans, tomatoes and seasonings then mix properly. Simmer for 5 minutes then add the rest of the veggies. You may add ¼ tsp of ground cumin, 2 cups of water, frozen tomatoes 2 tbsp of tomato paste.

4. Add corn then simmer for 30 to 60 minutes.

5. Add any veggies of your choice like chunks of sweet potato. Use fresh or frozen veggies but make sure you drain all canned veggies to lower the level of sodium.

6. Serve with baked tortilla strips and reduced fat cheese.

Nutritional Information: Calories: 204; Protein: 13 g; Fat: 7 g; Cholesterol: 26 mg; Sodium: 379 mg; Carbs: 24 g

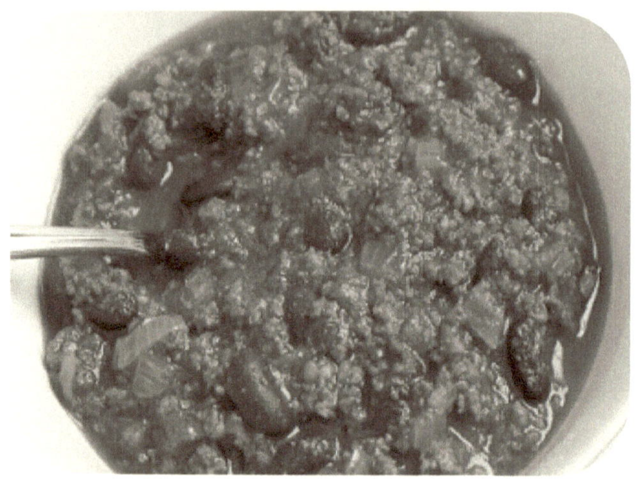

Bean Chili Soup

Roasted Squash Veggie Soup

Preparation time: 10 minutes

Cooking time: 50 minutes

Servings: 2

Ingredients:

1 butternut squash, chopped into cubes (or frozen butternut Squash cubes)

1 ½ cups of fresh spinach

2 tsp. canola oil, divided

1 cup of chopped celery

1 cup of chopped carrots

1 ½ cups chopped yellow onion

2 garlic cloves, finely chopped

1 tsp. of sage

3 cups reduced-sodium veggie broth

1 cup of water

½ tsp. nutmeg

Black pepper to taste

Directions:

1. Set the squash in a roasting pan then toss with 1 tsp of oil.

2. Roast for 40 minutes until brown at 400°F. Note that frozen squash may less time.

3. Once done, let it cool for some minutes then transfer to a blender and puree and then set it aside.

4. Pour the remaining oil into a large pot, add the veggies then sauté until soft over medium heat.

5. Pour in water, broth, spices, and the sautéed squash then simmer for 10 minutes. Serve.

Nutritional Information: Calories: 195; Sodium: 97 mg; Carbs: 38 g; Fat: 3 g; Cholesterol: 0 g; Protein: 4 g

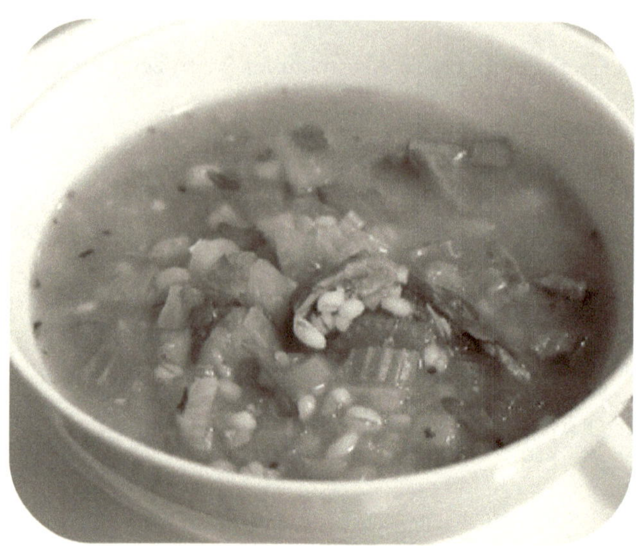

Beef Barley Soup

Slow Cooked Spiced Barley Beef Soup

Preparation time: 10 minutes

Cooking time: 8 hours

Servings: 4

Ingredients:

16.5 oz 75% lean ground beef, prepared

6.06 cups beef broth

2 cups brown/yellow onion

2 cups mushrooms

3 carrots

13.68 oz. barley

1 tsp dried thyme

1 tsp ground mustard

Powdered garlic

0.15 tsp Black Pepper

¼ tsp fine sea salt

Directions:

1. Brown beef then crumble into small pieces.

2. Add the rest of the ingredients, cover then cook for 8 hours on low.

Nutritional Information: Calories: 485, Fat: 14.81g; Cholesterol: 69.67mg; Sodium: 1103.5mg; Carbs: 62.36g

Caramelized Corn Veggie Soup

Preparation time: 15 minutes

Cooking time: 35 minutes

Servings: 12

Ingredients:

4 cups of corn kernels

6 cups veggie stock

1 ½ tbsp olive oil

2 cups diced carrots

3 cups of diced onion

2 cups of diced celery

1 tsp cumin

2 tsp diced garlic

¼ cup all-purpose flour

2 jalapeno peppers, finely chopped

1/8 tsp white pepper

1 ½ cups of half-and-half

1 tbsp diced parsley

1 tsp salt

Directions:

1. Heat up oven to 500°F then put the corn kernels on a baking sheet. Place in the oven and roast for 8 minutes until they start to caramelize.

2. Heat up oil in a large soup pot over medium-high heat. Add onion, garlic, celery, and carrots then cook for about 5 minutes, stirring frequently until the veggies are tender.

3. Lower heat then stir in the corn, cumin and flour. Stir until the flour evenly spread.

4. Pour in the veggie stock and jalapenos then simmer for about 30 minutes. Stir in parsley, pepper, half-and-half and salt. Remove from heat then serve.

Note: When you roast the corn, it develops its natural sugars and builds a caramelized flavor. You can use ½ tsp of cayenne pepper if you don't have jalapenos.

Nutritional Information: Calories: 119; Fat 5g; Cholesterol: 9 mg; Sodium: 184 mg; Carbs: 17g; Protein: 3g

Tomato Kale Sorghum Soup

Preparation time: 15 minutes

Cooking time: 1 hour

Servings: 10

Ingredients:

½ cup uncooked whole grain sorghum

12 oz. kale, stem removed, diced into 1 - 2" pieces

4 cups + 3 cups of chicken broth, divided (reduced-sodium)

2 (15 oz.) cans white kidney beans/cannellini, rinsed then drained

1 (15 oz.) can chopped tomatoes in juice

2 large garlic cloves, chopped finely (don't mince)

1 tbsp extra-virgin olive oil

¼ tsp of black pepper

1 small to medium onion, diced

1 tsp hot sauce or sriracha

¼ tsp of Kosher salt

Pecorino Romano cheese

Directions:

1. Boil three cups of broth then add ½ cup of sorghum. Boil gently for about 20 to 25 minutes. It's okay if the liquid still remains.

2. On the other hand, heat up a big saucepan, covered with its lid over medium to medium-high heat. Add olive oil then sauté onion, pepper, garlic and salt. Cook for about 6 to 8 minutes until the onion becomes tender.

3. Add the kale and hot sauce/sriracha then cook for 4 minutes until the veggie wilt.

4. Blend ½ cup of the white beans in a food processer or mash properly with the back of a fork or spoon.

5. Pour the blended beans, the rest of the whole beans, broth/sorghum mixture, canned tomatoes and extra 4 cups of reduced sodium chicken broth into the kale mixture.

6. Cover and bring to boil. Lower the heat to simmer for about 20 minutes.

7. Garnish each bowl with 1 tsp of grated parmesan cheese. Serve.

Nutrition Information: Calories: 175; Fat: 2 g; Sodium: 286 mg; Fiber: 9 g; Sugar: 2 g; Protein: 10 g

Dash Green Bean Soup

Preparation time: 10 minutes

Cooking time: 35 minutes

Servings: 9

Ingredients:

3 cups of chopped fresh tomatoes

1 lb. fresh green beans, cut into 1" pieces

1 cup of diced onion

1 cup of diced carrots

1 clove of garlic, finely chopped

2 tsp of butter

¼ cup finely chopped fresh basil (or 1 tbsp if dried)

6 cups of low-sodium veggie or chicken broth

¼ tsp of pepper

½ tsp of salt

Directions:

1. Sauté onion and carrots in butter in a large saucepan for 5 minutes. Pour in the broth, garlic and beans, stirring and bring to boil. Lower heat, cover then simmer for 20 minutes or until the veggies are soft.

2. Add the tomatoes, pepper, basil and salt; stirring, cover then simmer for another 5 minutes.

Nutritional Information: Calories: 58; Fat: 1g; Cholesterol: 2mg; Sodium: 535mg; Carbs: 10g; Protein: 4g

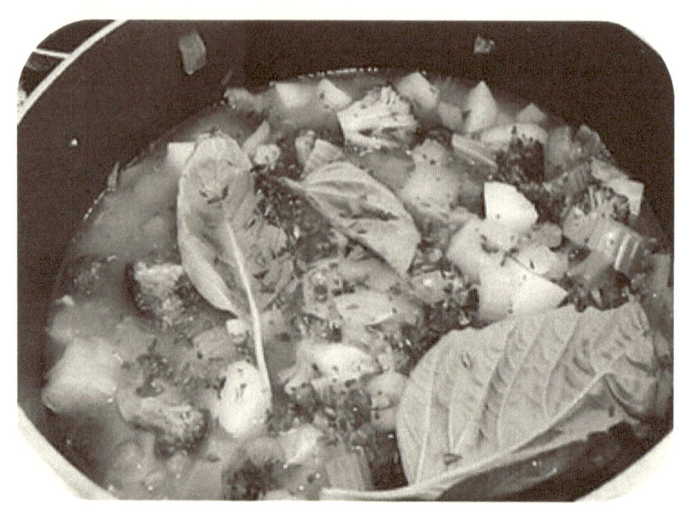

Veggie Soup

Dash Asparagus Veggie Soup

Preparation time: 20 minutes

Cooking time: 55 minutes

Servings: 12

Ingredients:

2 lbs. fresh asparagus, trimmed then sliced into 1" pieces

1 tbsp of butter

1 medium carrot, sliced thinly

1 tbsp of olive oil

1 medium onion, diced

6 cups of low-sodium chicken broth

¼ tsp of pepper

Low-fat sour cream, optional

¼ tsp dried thyme

2/3 cup long grain brown rice, uncooked

Salad croutons, optional

½ tsp of salt

Directions:

1. Melt butter and heat up oil in a 6-quart stockpot over medium heat. Stir in the veggies and seasonings, and cook for 8 to 10 minutes until the veggies are soft, stirring from time to time.

2. Stir in the broth and rice then bring to boil. Lower heat; simmer for 40 to 45 minutes, while the pot covered, until the rice is soft, stirring from time to time.

3. Use an immersion blender to puree the soup or you can allow the soup cool then puree in batches in a blender.

4. Return pureed mixture to the pot then heat properly. Serve with croutons and sour cream if desired.

5. Freezing option: Transfer soup to freezer containers then freeze. When ready to use, thaw a bit overnight in the refrigerator so the soup may separate. Reheat to boiling in a saucepan, whisking until it blends.

Nutritional Information: Calories: 79; Fat: 3g; Cholesterol: 3mg; Sodium: 401mg; Carbs: 11g; Protein: 4g

Spinach-Barley Turkey Soup

Preparation time: 10 minutes

Cooking time: 20 minutes

Servings: 6

Ingredients:

2 cups of cooked turkey breast cubes

2 cups of fresh baby spinach

2/3 cup quick-cooking barley

1 tbsp of canola oil

5 medium carrots, diced

6 cups low-sodium chicken broth

1 medium onion, diced

½ tsp of pepper

Directions:

1. Heat oil in a large saucepan over medium-high heat. Add the onion and carrots then cook for 4 to 5 minutes, stirring until the carrots are crisp-soft.

2. Stir in the broth and barley then bring to boil. Lower heat then simmer for 10 to 15 minutes while the pan is covered. Cook until the barley and carrots are soft. Stir in the turkey, pepper and spinach then heat properly.

Nutritional Information: Calories: 208; Fat: 4g; Cholesterol: 37mg; Sodium: 662mg; Carbs: 23g; Protein: 21g

Dash Veggie Beef Soup

Preparation time: 20 minutes

Cooking time: 55 minutes

Servings: 8

Ingredients:

1 ½ lbs. 90% lean ground beef

4 (14 ½ oz. each) cans low-sodium beef broth

1 ½ cups of shredded cabbage

¼ cup of tomato paste

5 oz. red potato, chopped finely (about 1 medium)

1 medium onion, diced

1 medium zucchini, roughly diced

2 garlic cloves, finely chopped

1(10 oz.) pkg. julienned carrots

1 tsp of dried basil

2 celery ribs, diced

1 (14 ½ oz.) chopped tomatoes, don't drain

½ tsp of dried oregano

½ cup frozen or fresh cut green beans

¼ tsp of pepper

¼ tsp of salt

Parmesan cheese, grated (optional)

Directions:

1. Cook beef, garlic and onion in a 6 quart stockpot for 6 to 8 minutes over medium heat until beef aren't pink anymore, crumbling the beef, then drain.

2. Add the celery and carrots, and cook, stirring for 6 to 8 minutes until soft. Stir in the tomato paste and cook for extra one minute.

3. Add the cabbage, tomatoes, green beans, zucchini, broth, potato and seasonings then bring to boil. Lower heat and simmer, covered for 35 to 45 minutes or until the veggies are soft.

4. Top with cheese if desired. Serve.

Nutritional Information: Calories: 207; Fat: 7g; Cholesterol: 57mg; Sodium: Carbs: 14g; Protein: 21g

Potato-Fennel Lemon Soup

Preparation time: 15 minutes

Cooking time: 25 minutes

Servings: 8

Ingredients:

2 large russet potatoes, peeled then sliced

2 tsp toasted fennel seeds

1 tsp of olive oil

2 lbs. fennel bulb, diced

2 tsp of lemon juice

1 cup of no-fat milk

3 cups low-sodium chicken broth

1 cup of diced red onion

Directions:

1. Heat up olive oil in a large soup pot over medium heat. Add the onion and fennel then sauté for about 5 minutes until the veggies are tender.

2. Stir in the chicken broth, potatoes, lemon juice and milk then cover and lower heat. Simmer for about 15 minutes until the potatoes are soft.

3. Puree the soup in batches in a blender until smooth. The soup will be hot, so in order to avoid burns, fill the blender no more than 1/3 of the soup.

4. Return the pureed soup to the pot then heat until it warms through.

5. Scoop soup into individual bowls then top with toasted fennel seeds. Serve at once.

Note: This recipe used no-fat cream instead of half-and-half cream and olive oil instead of butter to save 100 calories, fat of 1g, cholesterol of 37mg.

Nutritional Information: Calories: 149; Carbs: 28g; Sodium: 104mg; Fat: 1.5g; Cholesterol: 0.5g; Protein: 6g

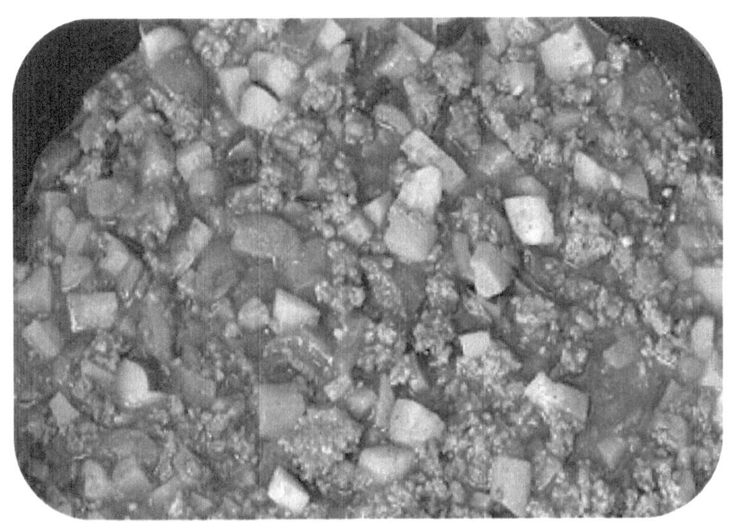

Creamy Avocado Zucchini Black Bean Tacos

Preparation time: 35 minutes

Cooking time: 2 minutes

Servings: 4

Ingredients:

For the salsa:

1 ½ cups of chopped tomatoes

Juice of 1 lime

½ cup of red onion

¼ tsp of salt

For the tacos:

8 corn tortillas

1 large grated zucchini

½ tsp powdered chipotle

1 (15 oz.) can black beans, rinsed

¼ tsp of paprika

½ tsp powdered chili

¼ tsp powdered garlic

For the avocado crema:

1 avocado, discard pit

Juice of 1 lime

½ cup reduced-fat Greek yogurt

¼ tsp of salt

Directions:

1. In a medium mixing bowl, combine black bean, grated zucchini and spices then toss to incorporate.

2. Heat up each side of corn tortillas for 15 seconds over high heat on gas stove or microwave for 10 seconds.

3. Distribute the zucchini/black bean mixture evenly among tortillas then serve with avocado crema and salsa.

4. To make the salsa; In a small bowl, mix tomatoes, lime juice, onion and salt then toss to combine. Serve with tacos.

5. To make the avocado crema; Scoop out the inside f the avocado into a blender then add lime juice, yoghurt and salt. Blend until creamy and smooth. Serve with tacos.

Nutritional Information: Calories: 245; Fat: 10 g; Carbs: 35 g; Protein: 9 g

Roasted Whole Grain Veggie Salad

Preparation time: 20 minutes

Cooking time: 50 minutes

Servings: 15

Ingredients:

3 cups of dry farro (or any whole grain of your choice)

3 cups broccoli florets, (1 head broccoli)

3 cups of cauliflower florets (1 head cauliflower)

2 onions, peeled then sliced into wedges

¼ tsp black pepper, freshly ground

2 tbsp extra virgin olive oil

1 cup diced hazelnuts

¼ tsp sea salt (for the veggies)

1 cup of dried cranberries

3 tbsp diced fresh parsley

¼ cup of lemon juice, (about 2 lemons)

2 lemons zest

½ tsp sea salt

¼ cup apple cider vinegar

½ cup extra-virgin olive oil

Directions:

1. Pour the farro into a large pot then cover with water by 2 inches. Boil then lower to a simmer.

2. Cook for approximately 50 minutes or until farro is soft. Drain off too much water then set aside to cool.

3. Preheat the oven to 450°F.

4. Combine olive oil, onion wedges, broccoli, cauliflower, pepper and salt then toss to incorporate.

5. Roast the veggies in the oven for 20 to 25 minutes until they are caramelized. Take it out from the oven then allow it cool.

6. In a glass measuring cup, pour in the lemon juice and zest then add extra apple cider vinegar to make quantity of vinegar and juice to ½ a cup. Season with sea salt then add ½ cup of extra virgin olive oil and whisk until combined.

7. Toss roasted veggies, farro cranberries, hazelnuts, vinaigrette and parsley together. Gently toss then serve at room temperature or cold.

Note: This salad can be kept in the refrigerator, covered for up to 3 to 5 days.

Nutritional Information: Per serving: 322 kcal cal., 16 g fat (2 g sat. fat), 137 mg sodium, 6 g fiber, 7 g sugar, 9 g pro.

Cheesy Zucchini Bow Tie Pasta

Preparation time: 5 minutes

Cooking time: 20 minutes

Servings: 4

Ingredients:

2 ½ cups (6 oz.) whole wheat bow tie pasta, uncooked

½ cup crumbled feta cheese

1 tbsp of olive oil

1 (15 oz.) can cannellini beans, rinsed then drained

1 medium sliced zucchini

1 (2 ¼ oz.) can chopped ripe olives, drained

2 ½ cups diced tomatoes, (about 2 large)

2 clove of garlic, finely chopped

¾ tsp of freshly ground pepper

Directions:

1. Cook the pasta according to the instructions on the package, drain, retaining ½ cup of the pasta water.

2. On the other hand, heat oil in a large skillet over medium-high Add zucchini and sauté for 2 to 4 minutes until crisp-soft.

3. Add the garlic and cook, stirring for 30 seconds. Stir in the olives, beans, tomatoes and pepper then bring to boil.

4. Lower heat then simmer, uncovered for 3 to 5 minutes until the tomatoes are soft, stirring from time to time.

5. Stir in the pasta and add enough pasta water as desired to add moisture. Stir in the cheese. Serve.

Nutritional Information: Calories: 348; Fat: 9g; Cholesterol: 8mg; Sodium: 394mg; Carbs: 52g; Protein: 15g

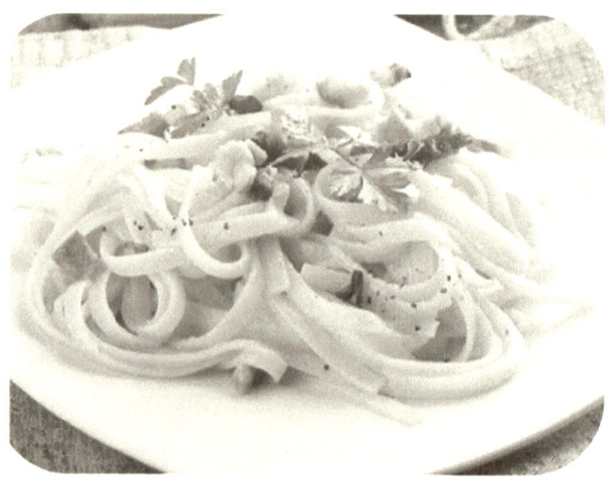

Pasta Dish

Cheesy Lentils 'N' Artichoke Sauce With Rice

Preparation time: 10 minutes

Cooking time: 25 minutes

Servings: 4

Ingredients:

1 (14 oz.) water-packed artichoke hearts, drained then diced

½ cup of dried red lentils, rinsed then sort

12 oz. (16 cups) diced fresh kale

¼ tsp dried oregano

1/8 tsp pepper

¼ tsp sea salt, divided

1 ¼ cups of veggie broth

2 tbsp grated Romano cheese

3 garlic cloves, finely chopped

1 tbsp grapeseed/olive oil

½ tsp Italian seasoning

2 cups basmati/brown rice, cooked and steamy

Directions:

1. In a small saucepan, combine red lentils, oregano, pepper, veggie broth and 1/8 tsp of salt then bring to boil.

2. Lower heat then simmer for 12 to 15 minutes, covered, until the lentils are soft and it has taken in almost all the liquid. Remove from heat.

3. Heat oil in a 6 quart stockpot, over medium heat. Add the kale and the rest of the salt. Cook for 4 to 5 minutes, covered, until the kale has wilted, stirring from time to time.

4. Add the garlic, artichoke hearts and Italian seasoning then cook, stirring for 3 minutes. 5. Remove from heat then stir in the cheese.

6. Serve kale and lentils mixture over rice.

Note: Lentils should be rinsed and sorted through for stones before cooking. You don't need to soak the lentils. Red lentils cook the fastest because they are split.

Nutritional Information: Calories: 321; Fat: 6g; Cholesterol: 1mg; Sodium: 661mg; Carbs: 53g; Protein: 15g

Green Soy Bean Kale Salad With Ginger Sesame Dressing

Preparation time: 15 minutes

Cooking time: 0 minute

Servings: 6

Ingredients:

10 oz. frozen shelled edamame, thawed (about 2 cups)

5 oz. baby kale salad blend (about 6 cups)

1 (15 oz.) can chickpeas/garbanzo beans, rinsed then drained

3 clementines, peeled then divided

½ cup of peanuts, salted

2 green onions, sliced diagonally

1 cup of fresh bean sprouts

½ cup of ginger sesame dressing

Directions:

1. Share salad blend among 6 bowls then garnish with the rest of the ingredients except salad dressing.

2. Serve with dressing. Enjoy!

Note: In Japan, green soy beans are known as Edamame which are boiled or steamed. Green onions should be sliced diagonally because it gives it a delicate appearance.

You can use navel orange if you don't have clementines or tangerines.

Nutritional Information: Calories: 317; Fat: 17g; Cholesterol: 0mg; Sodium: 355mg; Carbs: 32g; Protein: 13g

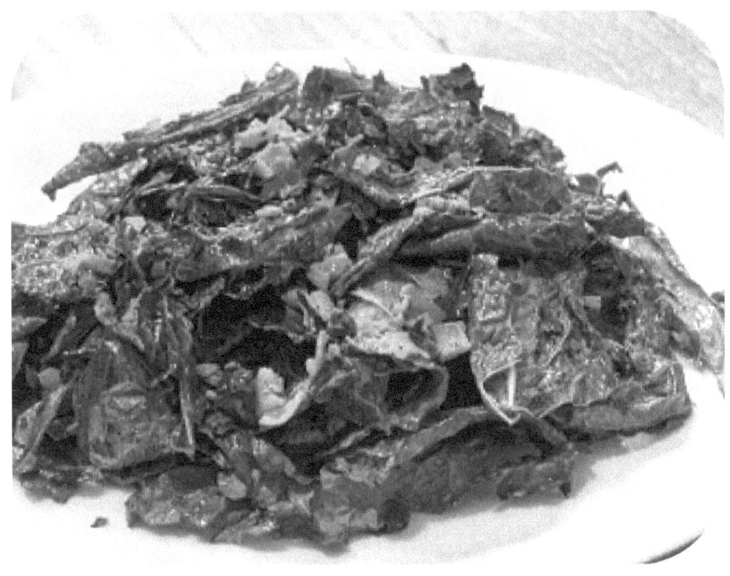

Kale Salad

Sweet Potato Black Bean Rice

Preparation time: 15 minutes

Cooking time: 35 minutes

Servings: 4

Ingredients:

1 large sweet potato, peeled then chopped

¾ cup of long grain rice, uncooked

1 (15 oz.) can black beans, rinsed then drained

¼ tsp of garlic salt

4 cups diced fresh kale, discard tough stems

1 medium red onion, minced

1 ½ cups of water

2 tbsp of sweet chili sauce

3 tbsp of olive oil, divided

Lime wedges (optional)

Extra sweet chili sauce (optional)

Directions:

1. In a large saucepan, combine rice, water, garlic and salt then bring to boil. Lower heat, then simmer, uncovered for 15 to 20 minutes or until the rice is soft and has taken in the water. Remove from heat then let sit for 5 minutes.

2. On the other hand, heat up 2 tbsp of oil in a large skillet over medium-high heat. Add the sweet potato and sauté for 8 minutes.

3. Add the onion and cook, stirring for 4 to 6 minutes until the potato is soft. Add the kale and cook, stirring for 3 to 5 minutes until soft. Stir in the beans and heat properly.

4. Stir in the rest of the oil and two tbsp of chili sauce gently into the rice. Add the potato mixture then serve with extra chili sauce and lime wedges if desired.

Nutritional Information: Calories: 435; Fat: 11g; Cholesterol: 0mg; Sodium: 405mg; Carbs: 74g; Protein: 10g

Creamy Lentil Medley

Preparation time: 15 minutes

Cooking time: 25 minutes

Servings: 8

Ingredients:

1 cup of dried lentils, rinsed

4 oz. crumbled feta cheese, (about 1 cup)

2 cups of water

1 medium cucumber, cut into cubes

2 cups of fresh mushroom slices

1 medium zucchini, cut into cubes

½ cup of diced soft sun-dried tomato halves

1 small red onion, diced

½ cup of rice vinegar

3 tbsp olive oil

¼ cup of finely chopped fresh mint

2 tsp of honey

1 tsp of dried basil

4 cups fresh baby spinach, diced

1 tsp of dried oregano

4 cooked bacon strips, crumbled (optional)

Directions:

1. In a small saucepan, boil the lentils with water. Lower heat then simmer covered for 20 to 25 minutes until soft. Drain then rinse in cold water.

2. Transfer the lentils to a big bowl then add tomatoes, zucchini, cucumber, mushrooms and onion.

3. Whisk oil, mint, vinegar, oregano and basil then drizzle this mixture over lentil mixture. Toss until well coated then add cheese and spinach.

4. Add bacon if desired then toss to mix. Enjoy!

Nutritional Information: Calories: 225; Fat: 8g; Cholesterol: 8mg; Sodium: 404mg; Carbs: 29g; Protein: 10g

Bulgur Tomato Garbanzo Tabbouleh

Preparation time: 5 minutes

Cooking time: 15 minutes

Servings: 4

Ingredients:

1 cup of bulgur

1 (15 oz.) can garbanzo beans or chickpeas, rinsed then drained

2 cups of water

5 oz. frozen or fresh peas, thawed (about 1 cup)

2 tbsp julienned soft sun-dried tomatoes

½ of cup finely chopped fresh parsley

¼ cup of finely chopped fresh mint

2 tbsp of lemon juice

¼ cup of olive oil

¼ tsp of pepper

½ tsp of salt

Directions:

1. Combine water and bulgur in a large saucepan then boil. Lower heat then simmer covered for 10 minutes.

2. Stir in peas then cook covered for 5 minutes until the peas and bulgur are soft.

3. Transfer to a big bowl then stir in the rest of the ingredients.

4. Refrigerate and serve cold or serve warm after cooking.

Note: The soft sun-dried tomatoes should not be soaked before using. Bulgur is whole grain that is made from boiled, dried and cracked whole wheat kernels.

Nutritional Information: Calories: 380; Fat: 16g; Cholesterol: 0mg; Sodium: 450mg; Carbs: 51g; Protein: 11g

Pintos 'N' Rice Salad

Preparation time: 5 minutes

Cooking time: 10 minutes

Servings: 4

Ingredients:

1 (15 oz.) can pinto beans, rinsed then drained

1 tbsp of olive oil

1 (8.8 oz.) pkg. brown rice, ready-to-serve

2 garlic cloves, finely chopped

1 cup of frozen corn

1 bunch romaine, quartered through the core lengthwise

1 small onion, diced

1 ½ tsp powdered chili

1 (4 oz.) can diced green chilies

1 ½ tsp of ground cumin

¼ cup cheddar cheese, finely shredded

½ cup of salsa

¼ cup diced fresh cilantro

Directions:

1. In a large skillet, heat oil over medium-high heat. Add corn and onion; cook and stir 4-5 minutes or until onion is tender. Stir in garlic, chili powder and cumin; cook and stir 1 minute longer.

2. Add beans, and then the rice, salsa, cilantro as well as the green chilies; heat and stir through, with occasional stirring.

3. Serve the dish over romaine wedges and then sprinkle with some cheese.

Nutritional Information: Calories: 331; Fat: 8g; Cholesterol: 7mg; Sodium: 465mg; Carbs: 50g; Protein: 12g;

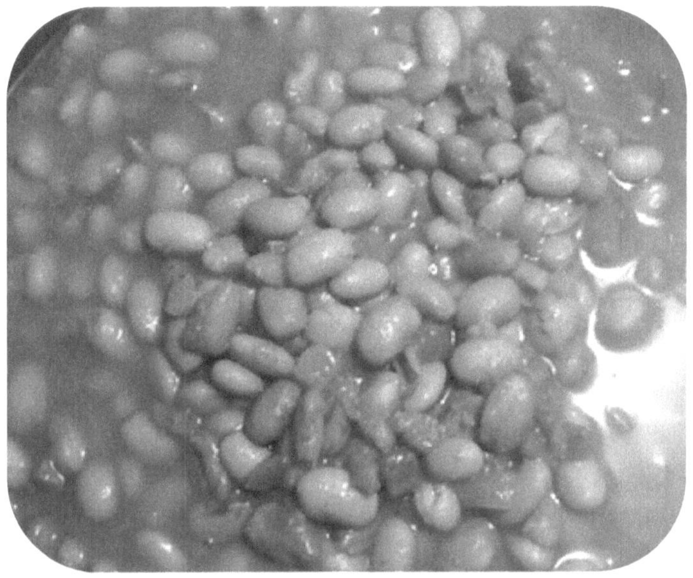

Pinto Beans

Dash Vegan Kebabs

Preparation time: 20 minutes (plus marinate time)

Cooking time: 40 minutes

Servings: 2

Ingredients:

½ cup of brown rice

1 cup of water

8 cherry tomatoes

1 small zucchini, cut into eight pieces

8 button mushrooms

1 red onion, sliced into four wedges

½ cup no-fat Italian dressing

1 green bell pepper, seed removed then sliced into four pieces

4 metal or wooden skewers (if wooden, soak in water for 30 minutes)

1 red bell pepper, seed removed then sliced into four pieces

Directions:

1. In a sealed plastic bag, combine zucchini, mushrooms, tomatoes, peppers and onion. Pour in the Italian dressing then shake the veggies to evenly coat them. Marinate the veggies for a minimum of 10 minutes.

2. Combine rice and water in a saucepan then heat over high heat. Boil then lower heat to low. Cover and simmer for 30 minutes or until the rice is soft and has taken in the water. Keep it warm in a small bowl.

3. Heat up a broiler or a gas grill or prepare a hot fire in a charcoal grill. Coat the broiler pan or grill rack lightly with cooking spray then place the cooking rack about 4 - 6" from the heat source.

4. Pass two tomatoes, two slices of zucchini, two mushrooms, one onion wedge, and one slice of red and green pepper through each skewer.

5. Set the kebabs on the broiler pan or grill rack or broiler pan. Sprinkle reserved marinade on top.

6. Broil or grill the kebabs for about 5 to 8 minutes, turning when required, until the veggies are soft.

7. Share the rice onto 2 plates then garnish with 2 kebabs. Serve at once.

Nutritional Information: Calories: 335; Fat: 3g; Cholesterol: 1mg; Sodium 335mg; Protein: 10g; Carbs: 67g

Southwestern One Bowl Veggies

Preparation time: 15 minutes

Cooking time: 1 hour

Servings: 6

Ingredients:

1 cup of cooked black beans

2 tsp of canola oil

½ cup of green lentils

1 cup diced red onion

4 lime wedges

1 tbsp fresh ground pepper

2 cups diced green bell pepper

1 chili pepper, finely chopped

½ cup of red lentils

2 garlic cloves, finely chopped

1 cup chopped sweet potato

2 tbsp finely chopped fresh cilantro

1 cup diced tomato

4 cups of diced kale

1 cup of brown rice

2 cups unsalted veggie stock

1 tbsp of ground cumin

2 cups of water

1 tbsp of red wine vinegar

Directions:

1. Heat up canola oil in a large sauté pan over medium-high heat. Add the onion, tomato, potato, garlic and peppers. Cook for 10 to 15 minutes, until the onions start to appear translucent.

2. Add the rice, stock, vinegar, spices, lentils and water then bring to a boil. Lower to simmer, cover and cook for 45 minutes.

3. Once done, toss with black beans, kale and cilantro then garnish with lime wedges. Serve.

Nutritional Information: Calories: 376; Fat: 4g; Cholesterol: 0mg; Sodium: 67mg; Carbs: 68g; Protein: 18g

Spring Veggies 'N' Rice Noodles

Preparation time: 10 minutes

Cooking time: 15 minutes

Servings: 6

Ingredients:

1 (8 oz.) pkg. rice noodles

1 tbsp of peanut oil

2 tbsp reduced-sodium soy sauce

1 tbsp of sesame oil

2 scallions, diced

1 tbsp of grated fresh ginger

2 garlic cloves, minced

1 cup of small broccoli florets

8 cherry tomatoes, halved

1 cup of fresh bean sprouts

1 cup diced fresh spinach

Red chili flakes, crushed (optional)

Directions:

1. Pour water into a large pot, about ¾ full then bring to a boil. Add the noodles then cook for 5 to 6 minutes until soft or according to instructions on the package. Drain then rinse properly with cold water. Set it aside.

2. Heat oils in a large frying pan or stockpot over medium heat. Add garlic and ginger then stir-fry until aromatic. Stir in broccoli and soy sauce and keep cooking for about 5 minutes over medium heat.

4. Add the rest of the veggies and cooked noodles then toss until properly warmed.

5. Share the noodles between warmed individual plates then garnish if desired with crushed red chili flakes. Serve at once.

Nutritional Information: Calories: 205; Fat: 5g; Cholesterol: 0mg; Sodium: 215mg; Carbs: 37g; Protein: 3g

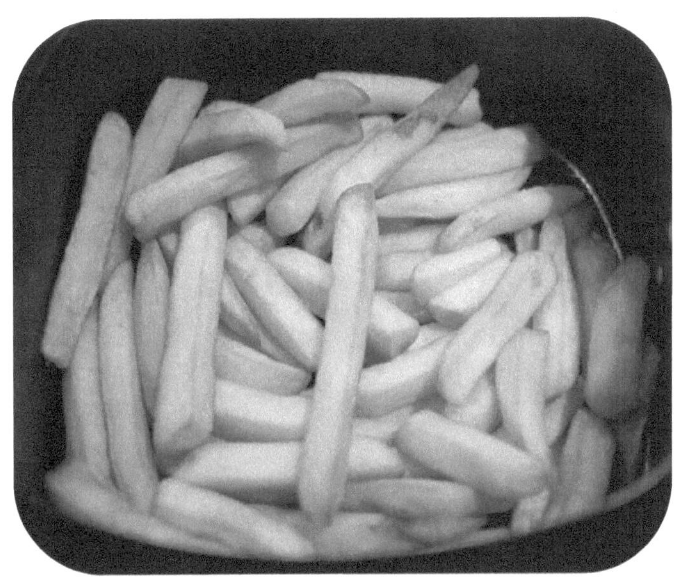

Creamy Roasted Cheesy Cauliflower

Preparation time: 5 minutes

Cooking time: 12 minutes

Servings: 6

Ingredients:

6 to 20 oz. frozen cauliflower florets

¾ cup low-fat Cheddar cheese, shredded

1 tbsp all-purpose flour

¾ cup no-fat milk

½ tsp of Dijon mustard

2 tbsp plain bread crumbs

1/8 tsp powdered garlic

Directions:

1. Stream fresh cauliflower for 8-10 minutes or cook according to instructions on the wrapper until soft then set aside.

2. In a small saucepan, whisk milk, garlic mustard and flour together until well combined.

3. Set over medium-high heat then simmer, stirring frequently. Lower heat and keep simmering, stirring gently for 2 minutes or until the mixtures thickens a bit.

4. Stir in cheddar cheese until it melt.

5. Preheat the broiler on high then assemble cauliflower in a baking pan then evenly pour cheese on top. Sprinkle bread crumbs on top then broil for 2 minutes or until the bread crumbs becomes golden brown.

Nutritional Information: Calories: 90; Fat: 3g; Sodium: 180 mg; Carbs: 9g; Protein: 6g

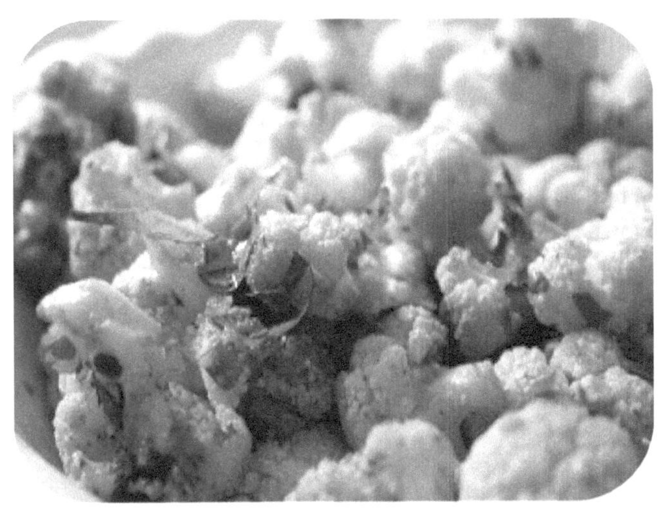

Fennel Tomato Bruschetta

Preparation time: 5 minutes

Cooking time: 10 minutes

Servings: 6

Ingredients:

½ whole-grain baguette, sliced into 6 (½" diagonal slices)

3 tomatoes, chopped

½ cup chopped fennel

1 tbsp of diced parsley

2 tbsp diced basil

1 tsp of olive oil

2 garlic cloves, finely chopped

1 tsp of black pepper

2 tsp of balsamic vinegar

Directions:

1. Place baguette slices in an oven and toast at 400°F until a bit browned.

2. Combine the remaining ingredients together then scoop equally over the toasted bread. Serve at once.

Nutritional Information: Calories: 110; Fat: 2 g; Carbs: 20 g; Protein: 3 g; Sodium: 123 mg

Chili Paprika Potato Wedges

Preparation time: 20 minutes

Cooking time: 30 minutes

Servings: 8

Ingredients:

3 large baking potatoes

1 ½ tsp powdered chili

3 tbsp olive or vegetable oil

1 ½ tsp of paprika

1 ½ tsp powdered onion

1 ½ tsp of powdered garlic

Directions:

1. Preheat the oven to 450°F.

2. Wash the potatoes by scrubbing properly but don't peel them.

3. Slice each potato into eight wedges, lengthwise.

4. Combine oil, chili, garlic, paprika and onion together then spread mixture on the sides of each potato wedge.

5. Set on a baking sheet creating space between each wedges.

6. Bake in preheated oven for 30 minutes.

Nutritional Information: Calories: 160; Fat: 6 g; Carbs: 25 g; Protein: 3 g; Sodium: 20 mg

Cheesy Whole Wheat Macaroni

Preparation time: 20 minutes

Cooking time: 40 minutes

Servings: 8

Ingredients:

1/3 cup shredded low-fat Cheddar Cheese

¾ lb. whole wheat elbow macaroni

2 ¾ cups no-fat milk

1 tsp no-salt-added butter

2 cups of panko breadcrumbs

1 ½ cups of low-fat shredded cheddar cheese

3 tbsp of all-purpose flour

1 tbsp of fresh thyme

2 tsp no-salt-added butter

1 cup of reduced-sodium chicken stock

2 tsp Dijon mustard

¼ tsp black pepper, freshly ground

1 tbsp of fresh thyme

Directions:

1. Preheat the oven to 400°F then coat a 3 qt shallow baking dish with butter.

2. Pour water into a large pot, about ¾ full then add a pinch of salt. Add the macaroni and cook until tender.

3. In a sauté pan, melt butter then add the panko breadcrumbs. Season with pepper and continue stirring over medium heat until it turns golden brown. Let it cool then add 1/3 cup of cheddar cheese until well mixed.

4. Melt butter in a large saucepan over low to medium heat then stir in flour for 3 minutes.

5. Stir in milk then bring to boil, whisking frequently then simmer. Whisk from time to time for 3 minutes. Stir in 1 ½ cup of cheddar, pepper, mustard and thyme, then remove from heat.

6. Stir chicken stock, macaroni and sauce together in a large bowl then transfer to the baking dish.

7. Baste cheese mixture and breadcrumbs evenly on top then bake in the center of the oven for 20 to 25 minutes, or until it becomes bubbling and golden.

Nutritional Information: Calories: 350; Fat: 8g; Carbs: 54g; Protein: 19g; Sodium: 360 mg

Mashy Creamy Cauliflower

Preparation time: 5 minutes

Cooking time: 5 minutes

Servings: 4

Ingredients:

8 cups cauliflower florets (about 1 medium head cauliflower)

1/3 cup fat-free plain sour cream/Greek yogurt

4 peeled garlic cloves

1 tsp of no-salt-added butter

Pepper to taste

½ tsp of salt

Directions:

1. In a micro-safe bowl, pour in the cauliflower florets then cover with a plate. Cook for about 3 to 5 minutes in the microwave without adding water until tender.

2. Drain then transfer to the blender, add butter, half of the yogurt and garlic, then puree until creamy and has slight lumps.

3. Pour in the remaining yogurt as required then add pepper and salt to taste.

Nutritional Information: Calories: 60; Fat: 1.3g; Carbs: 9g; Protein: 5g; Sodium: 342mg; Cholesterol: 2.7g

Roasted Hot Broccoli

Preparation time: 20 minutes

Cooking time: 25 minutes

Servings: 8

Ingredients:

8 cups broccoli slices (about 1 ¼ lbs. broccoli with large stems cut off and sliced into 2" pieces)

¼ tsp of crushed red pepper flakes

4 tbsp of olive oil, divided

¼ tsp black pepper, freshly ground

½ tsp unsalted seasoning blend

4 peeled garlic cloves, finely chopped

Directions:

1. Preheat the oven to 450°F.

2. Toss 2 tbsp of olive oil and broccoli in a large bowl then sprinkle pepper and seasoning on top.

3. Transfer to a baking sheet that has been rimmed then bake for 15 minutes.

4. On the other hand, combine red pepper flakes, garlic and 2 tbsp of olive oil.

5. Once the broccoli is cooked, ladle garlic oil all over the broccoli then shake the baking sheet to coat the broccoli.

6. Return to the oven then keep baking for about 8 to 10 minutes until the broccoli begins to brown. Serve immediately.

Nutritional Information: Calories: 86; Sodium: 24 mg; Fat: 7 g; Cholesterol: 0 mg; Carbs: 5 g; Protein: 2 grams

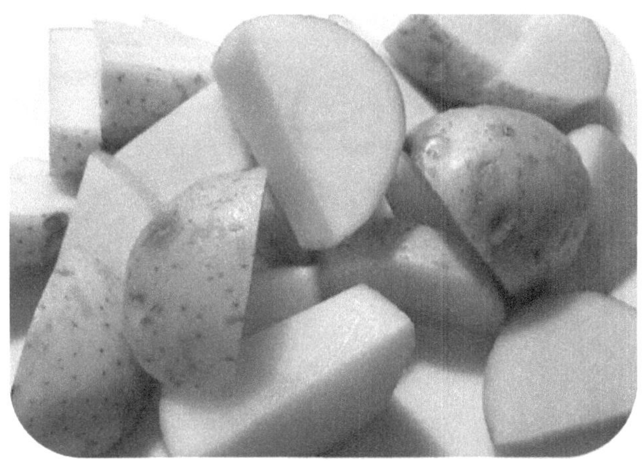

Seasoned Mashed Garlicky Potatoes

Preparation time: 20 minutes

Cooking time: 25 minutes

Servings: 8

Ingredients:

2 lbs. gold or red potatoes, scrubbed then sliced into chunky sizes

1 tsp unsalted seasoning blend

6 peeled garlic cloves

½ tsp black pepper, freshly ground

¼ cup of olive oil

Directions:

1. In a large saucepan, add the potato chunks and garlic then add cold water to cover and bring to boil.

2. Cook for about 25 minutes until soft a fork is pierced into it. Remove from heat.

3. Once done, drain off liquid, reserving ¾ cup of the potato liquid.

4. Add seasoning blend, olive oil, pepper and the reserved liquid. Mash with a big fork or a potato masher.

5. Taste then add more pepper and seasoning if desired.

Nutritional Information: Calories: 145; Sodium: 7 mg; Fat: 7 g; Cholesterol: 0 mg; Carbs: 19g; Protein: 2 g

Sweet Spicy Lime Pineapple

Preparation time: 9 minutes

Cooking time: 6 minutes

Servings: 6

Ingredients:

1 fresh pineapple

1 ½ tsp powdered chili

1 tbsp of olive oil

3 tbsp of brown sugar

1 tbsp of lime juice

1 tbsp agave nectar or honey

Dash of salt

Directions:

1. Peel the pineapple then take out the eyes. Slice into 6 wedges lengthwise and take out the core.

2. Mix the rest of the ingredients in a small bowl until well blended.

3. Rub half of the mixture all over the pineapple, keeping the remaining mixture for basting.

4. Broil the pineapple four inches from heat or grill each side over medium heat for 2 to 4 minutes until a bit browned, basting from time to time with the leftover glaze.

Nutritional Information: Calories: 97; Fat: 2g; Cholesterol: 0mg; Sodium: 35mg; Carbs: 20g; Protein: 1g

Zucchini Stuffed Turkey Pulp Sausage

Preparation time: 35 minutes

Cooking time: 20 minutes

Servings: 6

Ingredients:

6 medium (8 oz. each) zucchini

2 tsp dried basil (or 2 tbsp finely chopped fresh basil)

1 lb. Italian turkey sausage links, remove casings

2 medium tomatoes, seed removed then diced

1/3 cup of grated Parmesan cheese

1 cup panko bread crumbs

1/3 cup finely chopped fresh parsley

2 tbsp finely chopped fresh oregano (or 2 tsp if dried)

¾ cup of part-skim shredded mozzarella cheese

¼ tsp of pepper

Extra finely chopped fresh parsley (optional)

Directions:

1. Preheat the oven to 350°F. Slice each zucchini in half lengthwise then scoop out the pulp, you now have a ¼" shell. Chop the pulp.

2. Set the zucchini shells in a large microwave-safe dish then microwave in batches, covered for 2 to 3 minutes on high until crisp-soft.

3. Cook the zucchini pulp and sausage in a large skillet for 6 to 8 minutes over medium heat until the sausage isn't pink anymore, crumbling the sausage then drain.

4. Stir in breadcrumbs, herbs, cheese, tomatoes and pepper then scoop mixture into zucchini shells.

5. Place the stuffed zucchini in 2 ungreased 13 by 9" baking dishes then bake, covered for 15 to 20 minutes until soft.

6. Baste with mozzarella cheese then bake, uncovered for another 5 to 8 minutes until the cheese completely melt.

7. Sprinkle extra finely chopped parsley if desired.

Nutritional Information: Calories: 206; Fat: 9g; Cholesterol: 39mg; Sodium: 485mg; Carbs: 16g; Protein: 17g

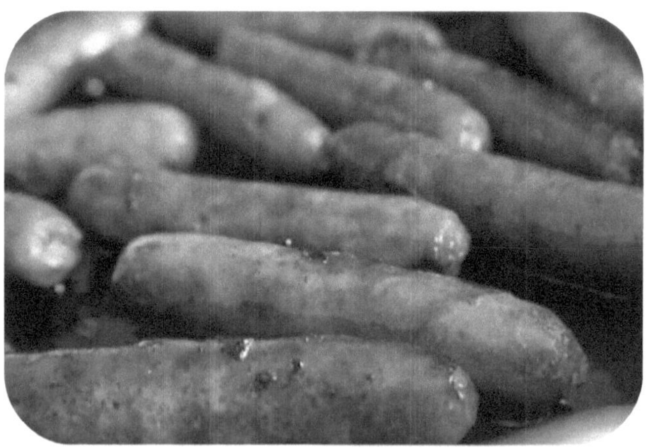

Sausages

Brown Rice Pistachio Pilaf

Preparation time:

Cooking time:

Servings: 8

Ingredients:

1 1/8 cups dark brown rice, rinsed then drained

3 tbsp of fresh orange juice

¼ cup diced pistachio nuts

¾ tsp of salt

½ tsp of grated orange zest

¼ tsp of ground turmeric or saffron threads

1 ½ tbsp of pistachio/canola oil

2 cups of water

¼ cup of diced dried apricots

Directions:

1. Mix water, rice, saffron and ¼ tsp of salt in a saucepan over high heat then boil.

2. Lower heat to low, cover then simmer for 45 minutes until the rice is soft and has absorbed the water. Transfer to a large bowl to keep warm.

3. Combine orange juice and zest, ½ tsp of salt and oil in a small bowl then whisk until well blended.

4. Pour the orange mixture over the rice then add apricots and nuts, and gently toss to coat. Serve at once.

Note: You can use any brown rice and pistachio oil adds flavor to the dish and gives it a rich taste.

Nutritional Information: Calories: 153; Fat: 5g; Carbs: 24g; Sodium: 222 mg; Cholesterol: 0 mg; Protein: 3g

Creamy Ginger Corn Pudding

Preparation time: 5 minutes

Cooking time: 20 minutes

Servings: 8

Ingredients:

2 cups polenta or coarse cornmeal

3 cups of water

1/8 tsp of ginger

3 cups of skim milk

¼ tsp cinnamon

1/8 tsp nutmeg

¼ cup maple syrup

1/8 tsp clove

½ cup of raisins

Directions:

1. Bring milk and water to a boil in a saucepan. Add the cornmeal then stir to remove lumps.

2. Boil again then lower heat to low, cover and stir from time to time for 10 to 15 minutes.

3. Turn off heat then stir in the rest of the ingredients. Let it rest for 10 to 15 minutes. Stir then serve with anything grilled.

Nutritional Information: Calories: 213; Fat: 1g; Cholesterol: 2 mg; Sodium: 44 mg; Carbs: 45g; Protein: 6

Dash Fresh Fruity Kebabs

Preparation time: 10 minutes

Cooking time: 0 minutes

Servings: 2

Ingredients:

4 (½" each) pineapple chunks

6 oz. lemon yogurt, no-sugar, low-fat

½ banana, sliced into 4 ½" chunks

1 tsp of fresh lime juice

4 strawberries

1 tsp lime zest

4 red grapes

1 peeled kiwi, quartered

4 wooden skewers

Directions:

1. Whisk the lime zest and juice and yogurt in a small bowl, cover then refrigerate until required.

2. Pass each of the fruit through the skewer. Do this with the other skewers until you've exhausted the whole fruits. Serve with lemon lime dip.

Note: You can use any kind of fruit including exotic fruits such as prickly pears, kumquats or star fruit. To avoid fruit browning, dip in orange or pineapple juice.

Nutritional Information: Calories: 190; Fat: 2g; Cholesterol: 5 mg; Sodium: 53 mg; Carbs: 39g; Protein: 4

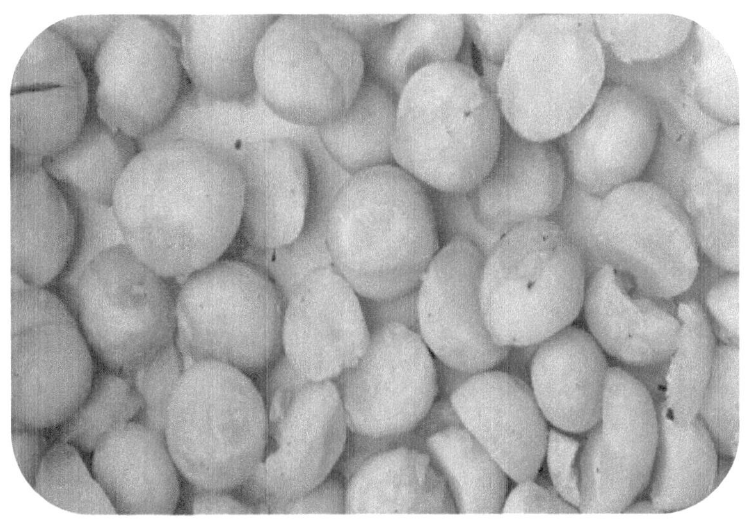

Apricot Soy Nut Mix

Preparation time: 5 minutes

Cooking time: 0 minutes

Servings: 5 cups

Ingredients:

1 cup of soy nuts, roasted

1 cup of dried apricots, diced

1 cup shelled pistachios, roasted

1 cup of raisins

1 cup of pumpkin seeds

Directions:

1. In a bowl, combine all the ingredients.

2. Spoon mix into ¼ cup sizes then place in a zip-top snack bag.

Nutritional Information: Calories: 198; Sodium: 4 mg; Fat: 11 g; Cholesterol: 0 mg; Carbs: 18 g; Protein: 11 g

Crumbly Edamame Salmon Cakes

Preparation time: 15 minutes

Cooking time: 8 minutes

Servings: 4

Ingredients:

13 oz. of flaked salmon, cooked (about 2 cups)

½ cup frozen edamame, thawed

¼ cup of whole-wheat panko or bread crumbs

1 tbsp peeled fresh ginger, finely chopped

2 large egg whites

Canola oil

1 scallion, minced, green and white parts

1 garlic clove, grinded through a press

1 tbsp minced fresh cilantro

For serving: Lime wedges

Directions:

1. Combine egg whites, garlic, cilantro, scallion, ginger, panko and salmon in a medium bowl.

2. Stir in edamame then mold into four (3 ½" wide) cakes. Transfer to a plate lined with waxed paper then refrigerate for 15 to 30 minutes.

3. Coat a large nonstick skillet with canola then heat over medium heat.

4. Add the salmon cakes then cook each side for 3 to 4 minutes until browned.

5. Turn the cakes over and cook for another 3 to 4 minutes. Serve at once with lime wedges.

Nutritional Information: Calories: 267; Fat: 1g; Sodium: 166 mg; Protein: 21g

Dash Multi Grain Veggie Tuna Sandwich

Preparation time: 15 minutes

Cooking time: 3 minutes

Servings: 2

Ingredients:

2 hearty multigrain bread slices

1 (5 oz.) can tuna packed in water, low-sodium, drained

2 tbsp of lemon juice, freshly squeezed

2 tbsp extra-virgin olive oil

2 tbsp fresh parsley, diced

1/3 cup of fresh arugula (or other greens)

2 green onions, sliced

¼ cup whipped cream cheese, reduced-fat

1/3 cup of cherry tomatoes, sliced

Black pepper

Directions:

1. Put the tuna in a medium-sized bowl then set aside. Combine lemon juice, green onion, oil pepper and parsley in another bowl then whisk to incorporate.

2. Pour 2/3 of the mixture into the tuna then mix properly.

3. Coat both sides of the bread light with some of remaining mixture using a pastry brush or spoon.

4. Grill the bread on a non-stick skillet over medium high heat until both sides are golden. Toss the rest of the oil with arugula.

5. To set sandwiches; On each slice of grilled bread, spread two tbsp of cream cheese then spread half of the tuna mixture on each slice, followed with half of the greens and half of the tomatoes.

Nutritional Information: Calories: 361; Fat: 22 g; Carbs: 18 g; Protein: 24g

Dash Spiced Spicy Almonds

Preparation time: 20 minutes

Cooking time: 20 minutes

Servings: 10

Ingredients:

2 ½ cups of almonds, unblanched

1 tbsp of sugar

½ tsp ground cinnamon

1 ½ tsp of kosher salt

¼ tsp of cayenne pepper

1 tsp of paprika

½ tsp ground cumin

1 tbsp of canola oil

½ tsp of ground coriander

Directions:

1. Combine all the ingredients except the almonds and oil in a small bowl. In a separate bowl, mix almonds and oil then sprinkle the spice mixture over the almonds and toss to coat properly.

2. Transfer coated almonds to a 15 by 10 by 1" baking pan lined with foil and greased with cooking spray.

3. Bake for 15 to 20 minutes at 325°F until a bit browned, stirring twice. Let it completely cool then store in an airtight container.

Nutritional Information: Calories: 230; Fat: 20g; Cholesterol: 0mg; Sodium: 293mg; Carbs: 9g; Protein: 8g

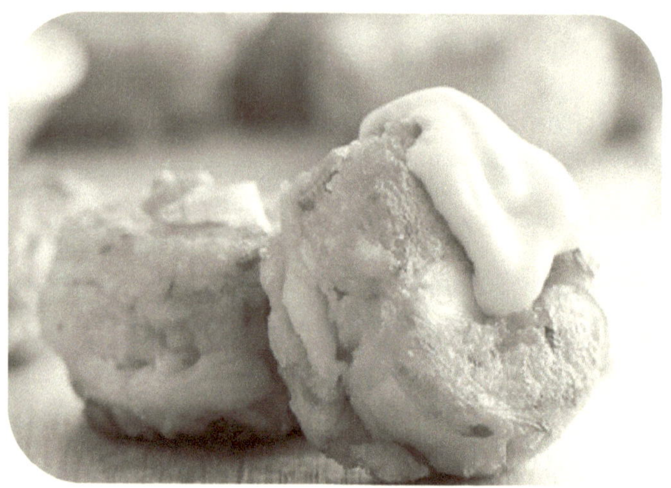

Mini Cakes

Lemon Beans Hummus

Preparation time: 5 minutes

Cooking time: 0 minutes

Servings: 10

Ingredients:

Pita breads, sliced into wedges

1 (15 oz.) can cannellini beans, rinsed then drained

2 peeled cloves of garlic

3 tbsp of lemon juice

¼ cup tahini

¼ tsp of salt

1 ½ tsp of ground cumin

2 tbsp finely chopped fresh parsley

¼ tsp red pepper flakes, crushed

Fresh assorted veggies

Directions:

1. Process garlic in a food processor until finely chopped then add pepper flakes, cumin, lemon juice, tahini, beans and salt. Cover then pulse until smooth.

2. Scoop puree into a small bowl then stir in parsley.

3. Refrigerate until you are ready serve. Serve fresh veggies and pita wedges. Enjoy!

Nutritional Information: Calories: 78; Fat: 4g; Cholesterol: 0g: Sodium: 114mg; Carbs: 8g; Protein: 3g

Banana Grain Pancakes

Preparation time: 10 minutes

Cooking time: 20 minutes

Servings: 8

Ingredients:

1 medium ripe banana, mashed (2/3 cup mashed)

1 cup of whole wheat flour

4 tsp of baking powder

1 cup all-purpose flour

½ tsp of salt

1 tsp of ground cinnamon

2 large eggs

1 tbsp of olive oil

2 cups no-fat milk

½ tsp of vanilla extract

1 tbsp of maple syrup

Banana slices + extra syrup (optional)

Directions:

1. In a bowl, whisk the flours, baking powder, cinnamon and salt together.

2. Whisk milk, eggs, oil, mashed banana, vanilla and syrup together in a separate bowl.

3. Pour the milk mixture into the flour mixture then stir until moistened.

4. Coat a griddle with cooking spray then preheat over medium heat.

5. Pour ¼ cupfuls of the mixture into griddle then cook until it starts to pop, bubbles appear on top and the bottoms turn golden brown.

6. Flip over and cook the other side until golden brown.

7. Serve with extra syrup and banana slices if desired.

8. To freeze; let the pancakes cool then freeze between layers of waxed paper in a re-sealable plastic freezer bag.

9. When ready to use; place the pancakes on an uncoated baking sheet then cover with foil. Preheat oven to 375°F then reheat pancakes for 10 to 15 minutes until well heated. You may also reheat by placing a stack of 2 pancakes in a micro-safe dish then microwave for 45 to 60 seconds on high until well heated.

Nutritional Information: Calories: 186; Fat: 4g; Cholesterol: 48mg; Sodium: 392mg; Carbs: 32g; Protein: 7g

Coconut Almond Oat Granola

Preparation time: 20

Cooking time: 1 hour 20 minutes

Servings: 8

Ingredients:

2 cups of almonds, roughly chopped

1 cup of shredded coconut, sweetened

2 chai tea bags

¼ cup olive oil

3 cups of quick-cooking oats

¼ cup of boiling water

1/3 cup of sugar

2 tsp of vanilla extract

¾ tsp of salt

¾ tsp of ground cinnamon

½ cup of honey

¼ tsp of ground cardamom

¾ tsp ground nutmeg

Directions:

1. Preheat the oven to 250°F. Steep the tea bags in boiling water for 5 minutes.

2. On the other hand, mix coconut, almonds and oats.

3. Throw away the tea bags then stir in the rest of the ingredients. Pour tea mixture into the coconut mixture then mix until well combined.

4. Spread batter evenly in an oiled 15 by 10" rimmed pan. Bake for 1 hour 14 miinutes, stirring at interval every 20 minutes, until it turns golden brown.

5. When done, let it completely cool without stirring then store in an airtight container.

Nutritional Information: Calories: 272; Fat: 16g; Cholesterol: 0mg; Sodium: 130mg; Carbs: 29g; Protein: 6g

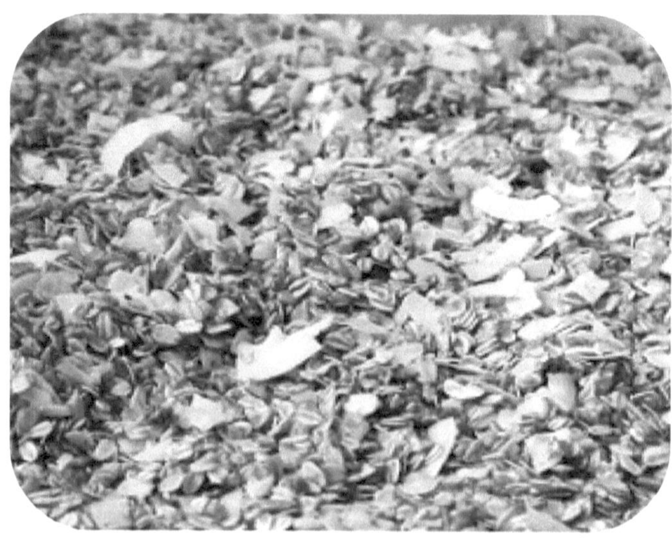

Sweet Almond Fruity Bites

Preparation time: 40 minutes plus chilling time

Cooking time: 0 minute

Servings: 48

Ingredients:

¼ cup of honey

3 ¾ cups almond slices, divided

1 cup minced dried cranberries or cherries

¼ tsp of almond extract

1 cup toasted chopped pistachios

2 cups of chopped dried apricots

Directions:

1. Pulse 1 ¼ cups of almonds in a food processor until finely chopped then transfer to a shallow bowl; kept for coating.

2. Pulse the rest of the almonds in a food processor until finely chopped. Add extract, while pulsing, add the honey slowly.

3. Transfer to a large bowl then, stir in cherries and apricots.

4. Share mixture 6 portions then mold each portion into a thick ½" roll. Wrap rolls in plastic then refrigerate 1 hour until set.

5. Remove wrap then slice rolls into 1 ½" sizes. Roll half of the rolls in kept almonds, gently pressing to stick. Roll the other half of the rolls in pistachios.

6. Wrap each roll in waxed paper if you like then twist the ends to seal.

7. If unwrapped, store in airtight containers, layered between waxed paper.

Nutritional Information: Calories 86; Fat: 5g; Cholesterol 0mg; Sodium; 15mg; Carbs: 10g; Protein; 2g

Crispy Tortilla 'N' Fruity Salsa Chips

This snack recipe is delicious, kid-friendly and easy to make.

Preparation time: 20 minutes

Cooking time: 12 minutes

Servings: 10

Ingredients:

For the fruit salsa:

3 cups chopped fresh fruits (like grapes, strawberries, kiwi, oranges, apples and other fresh fruits)

2 tbsp of orange juice

1 tbsp agave nectar or honey

2 tbsp no-sugar jam

For the tortilla crisps:

8 whole-wheat tortillas

½ tbsp of cinnamon

1 tbsp of sugar

Directions:

1. Preheat the oven to 350°F then slice each tortilla into ten wedges. Spread wedges on 2 baking sheets, ensure they aren't overlapped.

2. Grease the tortilla wedges with cooking spray.

3. Mix cinnamon and sugar in a small bowl then evenly sprinkle over the wedges.

4. Bake for 10 to 12 minutes until crisp. Transfer to a cooling rack then allow it cool.

5. Chop the fruit into cubes then mix the fruits gently in a mixing bowl.

6. Whisk orange juice, honey and jam together in a separate bowl. Pour juice mixture over the chopped fruits then gently mix.

7. Cover the bowl with a plastic wrap then refrigerate for 2 to 3 hours. Serve as topping for tortilla chips or as dip.

Nutritional Information: Calories: 119; Fat: 3g; Sodium: 90mg; Cholesterol: 0mg; Carbs: 21g; Protein 2g

Buttered Rosemary Crispy Potato Skin

Preparation time: 15 minutes

Cooking time: 1 hour 10 minutes

Servings: 2

Ingredients:

2 medium-size russet potatoes

1/8 tsp of black pepper, freshly ground

1 tbsp finely chopped fresh rosemary

Cooking spray, butter-flavored

Directions:

1. Preheat the oven to 375°F.

2. Scrub the potatoes then puncture with a fork. Set in the oven then bake for 1 hour until the skins are crisp.

3. Slice the potatoes in half carefully then spoon out the pulp. You now have 1/8" potato flesh stuck to the skin. Be careful as potatoes will be very hot. Reserve the pulp for later use.

4. Grease inside each potato skin cooking spray. Add the pepper and rosemary, pressing it in then bake for 5 to 10 minutes. Serve at once.

Note: You can use desired spices or herbs such as thyme, tarragon, garlic, cayenne pepper, dill to season potato skin.

Nutritional Information: Calories: 114; Fat: 0g; Cholesterol: 0mg; Sodium: 18mg; Carbs: 27g; Protein: 2g

Spicy Honey Pineapple Snack Mix

Preparation time: 15 minutes

Cooking time: 45 minutes

Servings: 12

Ingredients:

2 (15 oz. each) cans garbanzos, rinsed, drained then pat dry

1 cup of dried pineapple chunks

2 tbsp of honey

1 cup of raisins

2 cups of wheat squares cereal

½ tsp powdered chili

2 tbsp Worcestershire sauce

1 tsp powdered garlic

Butter-flavored cooking spray

Directions:

1. Heat the oven to 350°F. Grease a 15 ½ by 10 ½" baking sheet lightly with cooking spray.

2. Spray a heavy skillet with enough cooking spray then add garbanzos and cook for 10 minutes over medium heat, stirring constantly until the beans starts to brown.

3. Transfer garbanzos to the greased baking sheet then lightly spray beans with cooking spray.

4. Bake for 20 minutes, stirring constantly until crisp.

5. Grease the roasting pan lightly cooking spray then spoon cereal, raisins and pineapple into the pan. Add the roasted garbanzos and evenly mix.

6. Combine honey, spices and Worcestershire sauce in a big glass measuring cup. Stir to evenly mix then pour the mixture over the snack then gently toss.

7. Spray the mixture again with cooking spray then bake for 10 to 15 minutes, stirring from time to time to prevent the mixture from burning.

8. Take out from oven then allow it cool, and then store in an airtight container.

Note: Garbanzos and dried fruits were used in this recipe instead of pretzels and peanuts due to the increased amount of fiber and also low sodium and fat.

Nutritional Information: Calories: 194; Fat: 2; Cholesterol: 0g; Sodium: 218g; Carbs: 39g; Protein: 5g;

Pickled Peppercorn Asparagus

Preparation time: 15 minutes

Cooking time: 0 minute

Servings: 6

Ingredients:

3 cups (1 lb.) fresh asparagus, trimmed

8 whole black peppercorns

¼ cup of pearl onions

1 sprig fresh dill

¼ cup of white wine vinegar

2 whole cloves

¼ cup of cider vinegar

3 whole garlic cloves

1 cup of water

6 whole coriander seeds

¼ tsp red pepper flakes

Directions:

1. Cut off woody parts of the asparagus then slice spears into sizes that will fit into the jars.

2. Put sliced spears in colander, wash properly then drain. Trim then onions then combine all the ingredients in an air-tight container.

3. Keep in the refrigerator for up to four weeks.

Note: Sterilize the jars and lid before use. Do these by simmering them in water for 5 minutes then allow them cool to room temp.

Nutritional Information: Calories: 24; Fat: 0g; Cholesterol: 0g; Sodium: 5mg; Carbs: 4g

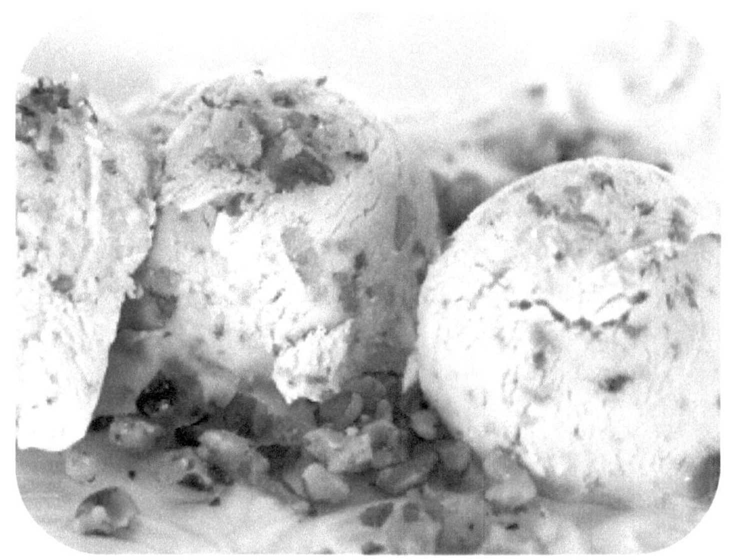

Spicy Ginger Turkey N Lettuce Wraps

Preparation time: 20 minutes

Cooking time: 30 minutes

Servings: 4

Ingredients:

1 lb. ground turkey, 93% lean

½ cup of instant brown rice

½ cup of water

1 tbsp finely chopped fresh ginger

2 tsp of sesame oil

1 large red bell pepper, chopped finely

½ cup of chicken broth, reduced-sodium

1 (8 oz.) can of water chestnuts, rinsed then diced

2 tbsp of hoisin sauce

½ cup diced fresh herbs (like chives, mint basil or cilantro)

1 tsp five-spice powder

½ tsp of salt

2 heads Boston lettuce, separate leaves

1 large shredded carrot

Directions:

1. In a small saucepan, boil water then rice; lower heat to low, cover then cook for 5 minutes. Take away from heat.

2. On the other hand, heat up oil in a large nonstick pan over medium-high heat then add the turkey and ginger. Cook for 6 minutes, using a wooden spoon to crumble until well cooked.

3. Stir in bell pepper, the cooked rice, spice powder, hoisin sauce, broth water chestnut, and salt then cook for a minute until well heated.

4. Share lettuce leaves among plates then scoop some of the turkey mixture into individual leaf. Garnish with carrot and herbs then roll.

5. To make ahead; make the filling, cover then refrigerate for a day. Reheat in microwave or serve chilled. Serve cold or reheat in the microwave.

Note: Tips: The Hoisin sauce can be refrigerated for a minimum of 1 year. Five-spice powder is considered a blend of Szechuan peppercorns, star anise, fennel seed, cloves and cinnamon.

Nutritional Information: Calories: 276; Fat: 10 g; Cholesterol: 65mg; Sodium: 595mg; Carbs: 21 g; Protein: 26 g

Soy Chocó Banana Cake
Preparation time: 30 minutes

Cooking time: 25 minutes

Servings: 18

Ingredients:

¼ cup powdered cocoa, unsweetened

½ cup mashed ripe banana (1 large one)

½ cup semisweet dark chocolate chips

½ cup brown sugar blend

2 cups all-purpose flour

¾ cup of soy milk

½ tsp of baking soda

1 large egg

¼ cup of canola oil

1 tbsp lemon juice

1 egg white

1 tsp vanilla extract

Directions:

1. Preheat oven to 350°F.

2. Grease an 11 by 7" brownie pan with nonstick spray.

3. In a large bowl, whisk cocoa, brown sugar, flour and baking soda.

4. In a separate bowl, whisk oil, egg, soy milk, egg white, bananas, vanilla and lemon juice.

5. Create a hole in the center of the flour mixture then pour in the wet mixture including the chocolate chips.

6. Stir everything together with a wooden spoon until combined then scoop batter into pan.

7. Bake for 25 minutes until the middle of the cake bounces back when lightly pressed with fingertips.

Nutritional Information: Calories: 150; Fat: 1g; Cholesterol: 12mg; Sodium: 52mg; Carbs: 27g; Protein 3g

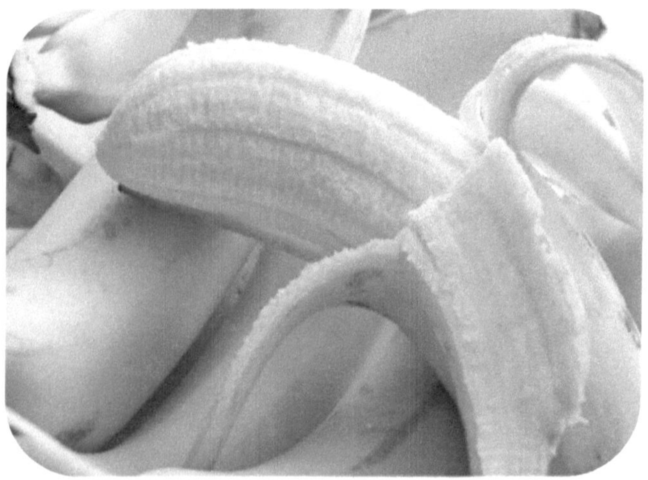

Dash Grainy Banana Bread

This delicious dessert bread is low in sodium and very healthy.

Preparation time: 20 minutes

Cooking time: 60 minutes

Servings: 14

Ingredients:

2 cups of mashed banana

½ cup of brown rice flour

¾ cup egg whites or substitute

½ cup of amaranth flour

2 tbsp of grapeseed oil

1 tsp baking soda

½ cup raw sugar

½ cup millet flour

½ tsp baking powder

½ cup of quinoa flour

1/8 tsp of salt

Directions:

1. Preheat the oven to 350°F. Lightly spray a 5 by 9" loaf pan with cooking spray then coat with small amount of any of the flours. Set it aside.

2. In a large bowl, combine all the dry ingredients except sugar. In another bowl, mix mashed banana, oil, egg and sugar then whisk to combine.

3. Pour the wet mixture into the dry ingredients then mix until well combined. Scoop batter into loaf pan then bake for 50 to 60 minutes.

4. Check if it's ready by sticking a toothpick into the bread. It's ready if the toothpick comes out clean. Take out the bread from the oven, allow it cool then slice. Serve.

Nutritional Information: Calories: 150; Fat: 3g; Sodium 150mg; Protein 4g;

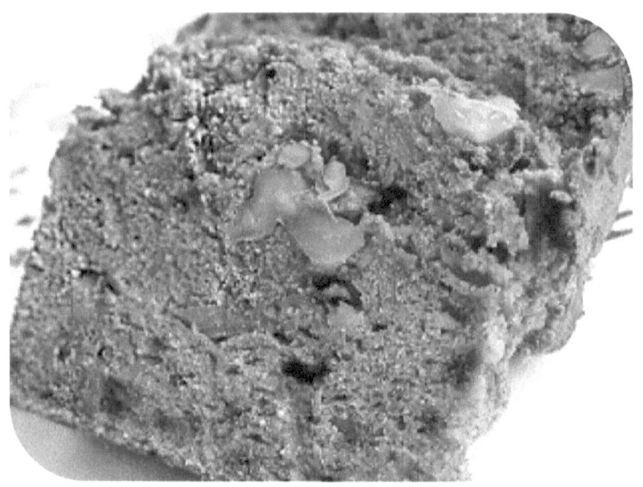

Chocolate Milk Pudding

Preparation time: 30 minutes

Cooking time: 0 minutes

Servings: 4

Ingredients:

1/3 cup chocolate chips

3 tbsp of cornstarch

2 tbsp of cocoa powder

2 cups fat-free milk

2 tbsp sugar

½ tsp of vanilla

1/8 tsp salt

Directions:

1. Combine cocoa powder, cornstarch, salt and sugar in a medium saucepan then mix until it incorporates.

2. Stir in milk and whisk, then heat up over medium, stirring from time to time until it becomes thick and bubbling.

3. Take off from heat then stir in vanilla and the chocolate chips until the chips melt and you have a smooth pudding.

4. Pour pudding into for individual dishes then refrigerate until set.

Note: Place a plastic wrap on top of the pudding to avoid a skin from forming.

Nutritional Information: Calories: 197; Fat: 5 g; Sodium: 138mg; Carbs: 31 g; Protein: 6g

Dash Cheesy Whole Grain Bruschetta

Preparation time: 20 minutes

Cooking time: 8 minutes

Servings: 4

Ingredients:

1 cup of ricotta cheese, low-fat

½ cup of Pomegranate Arils

6 whole grain nut bread slices

2 tsp fresh thyme

½ tsp of grated lemon zest

¼ tsp of sea salt (optional)

Directions:

1. Preheat the oven to 425°F. Set the slices of bread on a big baking sheet then bake for 8 minutes until a bit toasted.

2. Mix lemon zest and ricotta in a small bowl then top each toast with the lemon/ricotta mixture.

3. Sprinkle thyme and pomegranate arils on top.

Nutritional Information: Calories: 257; Fat: 6g; Cholesterol: 15mg; Sodium: 383mg; Carbs: 39g; Protein: 13g

Chocó Banana Mint Ice Cream

Preparation time: 15 minutes

Cooking time: 0 minute

Servings: 4

Ingredients:

3 tbsp of cocoa powder, unsweetened

3 bananas

½ tsp of peppermint extract

Directions:

1. Cut the bananas into slices the freeze.

2. Take out the banana slices from the freezer then thaw for about 5 minutes.

3. Pour the slices of bananas, peppermint and cocoa into a food processor then pulse until well chopped. Now puree until your mixture looks like a soft ice cream.

Note: Freeze the ice cream for some minutes if it becomes too soft after pureeing. Let the ice cream become firm then serve.

Nutritional Information: Calories: 99; Fat: 0g; Cholesterol: 0mg; Sodium: 1mg; Carbs: 22g; Protein: 2g

Dark Sautéed Rum Bananas

Preparation time: 20 minutes

Cooking time: 15 minutes

Servings: 6

Ingredients:

4 (1 lb) firm bananas

For the sauce:

2 tbsp dark rum/apple juice

1 tbsp of butter

2 tbsp brown sugar, firmly packed

1 tbsp canola/walnut oil

3 tbsp 1% low-fat milk

1 tbsp of honey

½ tsp canola oil

1 tbsp golden/dark raisins

Directions:

1. In a small saucepan, melt butter over medium heat.

2. Add honey, sugar and walnut oil then whisk, cooking and stirring constantly for about 3 minutes until the sugar completely dissolve.

4. Add milk, stirring in one tbsp at a time then keep cooking, stirring constantly for about 3 minutes until the sauce thickens a bit.

5. Take off from heat then stir in the raisins. Set it aside then keep it warm.

6. Peel the bananas then slice into three sections crosswise. Slice each section in half lengthwise then grease a big nonstick frying pan lightly with canola oil.

7. Set the pan over medium-high heat then add the banana slices. Sauté for 3 to 4 minutes until it starts to brown. Transfer to a plate then keep warm.

8. Pour rum into the pan then boil and deglaze the pan. Scrape any browned bit from the base of the pot by stirring with a wooden spoon. Cook for about 30 to 45 seconds until it reduces by half.

9. Return the banana slices to the pan then warm again.

10. Share banana slices among each bowls then ladle warm sauce on top then serve at once.

Note: Walnut oil gives the dish an exotic look and caramel sauce makes it sweet. Use apple juice instead of rum for non-alcoholic version.

Nutritional Information: Calories: 145; Fat: 6g; Cholesterol: 5mg; Sodium: 22mg; Carbs: 24g; Protein: 1g

Creamy Coconut Fruit Dessert
Preparation time: 10 minutes

Cooking time: 0 minute

Servings: 4

Ingredients:

½ of cup plain yogurt, no-fat

4 oz. softened cream cheese, no-fat

1 (8.25 oz.) can sliced peaches, water-packed, drained

4 tbsp toasted shredded coconut

1 (11 oz.) can mandarin oranges, drained

1 tsp of sugar

1 (8 oz.) canned pineapple chunks, water-packed, drained

½ tsp of vanilla

Directions:

1. Combine vanilla, sugar, yogurt and cream together in a small bowl then mix with an electric mixer on high speed until smooth.

2. Combine pineapple, peaches and oranges in another bowl then pour in the vanilla mixture, and then mix. Cover then refrigerate until completely chilled.

3. Transfer to individual bowls then top with shredded coconut and serve at once.

Note: Mandarin oranges are great source of vitamin A

Nutritional Information: Calories: 154; Fat: 2g; Cholesterol: 3mg; Sodium: 215mg; Carbs: 27g; Protein 7g

Oat Nut 'N' Fruity Bar

This dash dessert treat is a sweet treat and is a lot healthier than your everyday candy bar.

Preparation time: 10 minutes

Cooking time: 20 minutes

Servings: 24

Ingredients:

½ cup of oats

¼ cup of diced dried pineapple

½ cup of quinoa flour

¼ cup of flax meal

¼ cup buckwheat honey

¼ cup of wheat germ

¼ cup diced dried figs

¼ cup diced almonds

2 tbsp of cornstarch

¼ cup of dried apricots

Directions:

1. Mix all the ingredients then spread the mixture ½" thick over a sheet pan lined with parchment.

2. Bake for 20 minutes at 300°F then completely cool and sliced.

Nutritional Information: Calories: 61; Fat: 1g; Cholesterol: 0mg; Sodium: 5mg;

Mangarine Oat Peach Crumble

Preparation time: 20 minutes

Cooking time: 30 minutes

Servings: 8

Ingredients:

½ cup whole-wheat flour

8 ripe peaches, peeled, pit removed then sliced

¼ cup of uncooked quick-cooking oats

2 tbsp margarine, trans free, sliced into thin slices

3 tbsp lemon juice (juice from a lemon)

¼ tsp of ground nutmeg

1/3 tsp of ground cinnamon

¼ cup of dark brown sugar, packed

Directions:

1. Preheat the oven to 375°F. Grease a 9" pie pan with cooking spray.

2. Assemble the slices of peach in the oiled pie pan then sprinkle nutmeg, cinnamon and lemon juice on top.

3. Combine sugar and flour in a small bowl, whisking everything together. Crumble the margarine with your fingers into the sugar/flour mixture.

4. Pour in the uncooked oats then stir to evenly combine. Sprinkle flour mixture over the peaches.

5. Bake for about 30 minutes until the peaches are tender and the top is browned. Slice the peaches into eight equal slices then serve warm.

Note: Use freestone peaches for this recipe.

Nutritional information: Calories: 152: Fat: 4g; Cholesterol: 0mg; Sodium: 41mg; Carbs: 26g; Protein: 3g

Fruity Berries Ice Pops

Preparation time: 1 hour 10 minutes (plus freezing time)

Cooking time: 0 minutes

Servings: 6

Ingredients:

2 cups of apple juice, or desired juice

1 ½ cups chopped watermelon, cantaloupe and strawberries

6 (6 to 8 oz. each) paper cups

½ cup of blueberries

6 craft sticks

Directions:

1. Combine all the fruits together then share equally among the paper cups then pour 1/3 cup of juice into each paper cup.

2. Set the paper cups on a leveled space in the freezer then freeze for about an hour until half frozen.

3. Dip a craft stick into the middle of the pop then freeze until set/freeze.

Nutritional Information: Calories: 60; Fat: 0g; Cholesterol: 0mg; Sodium: 6mg: Carbs: 14g; Protein: 0.5g

Spiced Creamy Squash Potato Pie

Preparation time: 20 minutes

Cooking time: 55 minutes

Servings: 8

Ingredients:

1 (9") pre-made pie shell, frozen

1 (¼ lb) peeled sweet potato, cooked

½ cup of soy milk

1 (2 ½ lbs.) peeled buttercup squash, deseeded then cooked

¼ cup of egg whites

½ cup of silken tofu

¼ cup of rye flour

1 tsp grated fresh ginger

½ tsp each of ginger clove, vanilla extract, nutmeg and cinnamon

3 tbsp of honey

1 tsp of orange zest

Directions:

1. Heat up the oven to 300°F.

2. In a food processor, puree squash and sweet potato then transfer to a big bowl. Add the rest of the ingredients then stir until smooth and well-mixed.

3. Set the pie shell on a sheet pan then scoop mixture into each pie shell then bake for 45 to 55 minutes until the inner temp gets to 180°F.

Note: Rye flour tangy taste complements the filling sweet taste.

Nutritional Information: Calories: 210; Fat: 6g; Cholesterol: 0mg; Sodium: 109mg; Carbs: 34g; Protein: 5g

Dark Balsamic Strawberry Sorbet
This sorbet is packed with vitamin C and a classic Italian dessert for your parties.

Preparation time: 30 minutes

Cooking time: 5 minutes

Servings: 4

Ingredients:

1 tbsp of dark honey

4 cups hulled strawberries, halved + 4 berries, roughly diced

¾ cup of balsamic vinegar

Directions:

1. Simmer vinegar in a small non-aluminum saucepan over medium-low heat. Cook for approximately 5 minutes until it reduces by half then take away from heat and then allow it cool.

2. Process halved strawberries in a blender until completely smooth then pass it through a fine-mesh sieve set on top of a bowl; pressing on the solids firmly with the back of a wooden spoon or a rubber spatula collect all its juice.

3. Throw away the solids then pour honey and the reduced balsamic to the extracted juice.

4. Stir, cover then refrigerate until chilled.

5. Freeze according to the maker's directions. Keep in the freezer for up to 2 days or until ready to serve.

6. Scoop sorbet into serving bowls then top with diced strawberries.

Nutritional Information: Calories: 92; Fat: 0g; Cholesterol: 0mg; Sodium: 2mg; Carbs: 22g; Protein: 1g

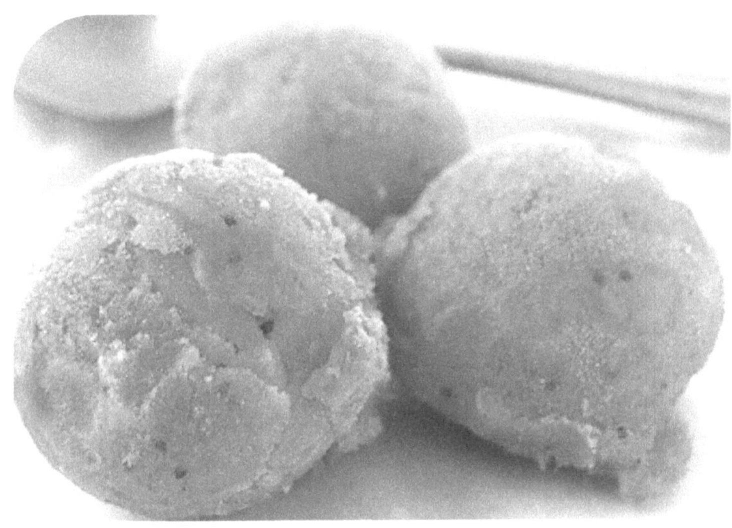

Strawberry Sorbet

The End